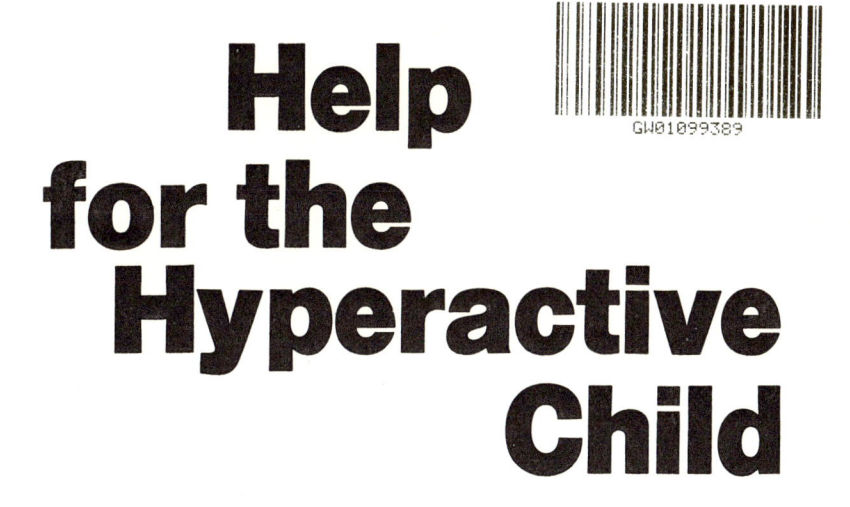

# Help for the Hyperactive Child
## through Diet and Love

Janey Walls Mitchell

Betterway Publications, Inc.
White Hall, Virginia

First Printing: September, 1984
Published by Betterway Publications, Inc.
  White Hall, VA 22987
Cover design by Albert DeRose
Typography by East Coast Typography, Inc.

© 1984 by Janey Walls Mitchell

All rights reserved. No part of this book may be reproduced by any means, except by a reviewer who wishes to quote brief excerpts in connection with a review in a magazine or newspaper.

**Library of Congress Cataloging in Publication Data**

Mitchell, Janey Walls,
    Help for the hyperactive child — through diet and love.

    Bibliography: p.
    Includes index.
    1. Hyperactive children.   2. Food allergy in children —
Diet therapy.   I. Title.
RJ506.H9M58   1984      618.92'8589      84-14573
ISBN 0-932620-40-X (pbk.)

Printed in the United States of America

To Harris, who tested my courage, my patience, my faith, and above all, my love.

In my anguished quest for answers, understanding, and guidance, my courage grew stronger, my patience grew more enduring. My faith was not destroyed but strengthened; my love did not fail, but grew more steadfast.

Through our storms, we emerged winners. Our story echoes triumphantly.

The word "he" throughout this book is meant to mean he or she. I chose deliberately to use it because more boys are hyperactive than girls, and for the sake of simplicity in writing this book.

# Contents

**Foreword** by Lendon H. Smith, M.D. .......................... 7
**Introduction** by the Author ................................. 9

## PART I: Our Ultimate Triumph

1. The Bubble Burst .......................................... 13
2. Child Renewal ............................................. 20

## PART II: On the Road to Success

3. Sweep Away Guilt .......................................... 27
4. From Rock Bottom .......................................... 31
5. Reinforcements ............................................ 39
6. Snack, Crackle, Flop ...................................... 44
7. Forward Movement .......................................... 53
8. Newsworthy Label .......................................... 65
9. Diet Diary ................................................ 69
10. Food: Friend or Foe? ..................................... 74
11. Food for a New Beginning ................................. 83

## PART III: Establishing a Balance

12. Our Supplement Friends ................................... 93
13. Essential Fatty Acids .................................... 102
14. Hair Can Talk ............................................ 104

## PART IV: Coping with an "Impossible" Child

15. No One Answer ............................................ 111
16. Smothering With Drugs .................................... 114
17. Unwind the Roller Coaster ................................ 122
18. Characteristic Pattern ................................... 131
19. Tackling Bad Habits ...................................... 144
20. Grapevine of Techniques .................................. 151

# PART V: Morsel Tips and Recipes

21. Yuk to Yum Morsels ...................................... 167
22. Helpful Tips ................................................ 169
23. Quick and Easy Recipes ................................ 171
Appendix A: The Natural Way Program ...................... 177
Appendix B: The Vitamin Alphabet ........................... 181
Appendix C: Minerals are Essential ........................... 191
Appendix D: Summary of Contributing Factors ............... 200
Appendix E: Glossary ........................................... 202
Appendix F: Suggested Reading ............................... 206
Appendix G: References ........................................ 209
Index ........................................................... 213

---

The information presented in this book has been prepared thoughtfully and carefully. However, it is not intended to be prescriptive or diagnostic. Readers are asked to use their own good judgment and to consult a health care professional when considering treatment of a child who may be hyperactive.

# Foreword

Although medical doctors are reluctant to believe that diet has anything to do with behavior, any reasonably aware parent, teacher, flight attendant, police person, counselor, minister, or sibling has long been aware of the connection between the ingestion of sugary non-foods and wild and inappropriate activity. I suspect that since heredity plays some role in the etiology of hyperactive behavior, children of doctors may not be as prone to the condition, and thus may be less aware of the problem as parents. Doctors need a long attention span to get through medical school, and the tendency toward uncontrollable restlessness may be rare among them and their families. Not personally familiar with it, the physician-parent may not believe the condition is common, making him less likely to believe the patient's parents who report this pathological restlessness.

Consequently, parents may feel guilty when they bring "the wild and restless" into the physician's office to get an answer. The doctor tends to suggest by his body language and often silent condemnation that if the parents had been more swift and sure with discipline all this could have been avoided. If the doctor could only find lead poisoning or anemia, worms or an infection or an allergy to explain the child's antics. But . . . nothing.

Hope lies ahead. The reader of this book will find it. With her simple, clear, linear, and cogent style Janey Walls Mitchell has been able to describe this type of child and to remove some of the onus of guilt from the shoulders of conscientious parents.

We all know we are supposed to give our children a good self image; an adult with a poor self-image is an incomplete human. As the child is growing we must show praise, acceptance, pride, and love — teach some rules and self-restraint. But how on earth can we do that if everything the child does is antisocial, dangerous, irritating, inappropriate or, at best, challenging? These children sabotage our efforts to civilize them. Everything we say to them is a command or a demand.

Janey has figured out the ways to communicate with difficult children. She has found ways to get the child to use his social brain, not the selfish, animal brain (the Devil in all of us).

It is easier to say nice things to a child who is cheerful and compliant. A happy child usually feels good. He feels good because he is eating the foods that nourish the social part of the brain.

I applaud Janey. She believes in the things I do. She is obviously an intelligent, thoughtful person.

Lendon H. Smith, M.D.<br>
Portland, Oregon

# Introduction

In the midst of despair, many parents are interested in starting their children on new diets to improve behavior. But they don't know where or how to start. That is why this book was written — to show parents of hyperactive and/or learning-disabled children how I made a new, happy boy of my son through diet modification.

A child's behavior, I discovered, can be improved by changing his diet. Medical research shows that what a child eats could be causing misbehavior, and that through a change of diet, he can be healthy, happy, and calm. Before I started my detective work, however, I was skeptical, in spite of all the research. I thought it was a hopeless waste of time to search for a solution to my child's problems.

Your experience may not be exactly the same, but perhaps you will be able to identify with me in my struggle to help my son. Whether your child's problems are few or many, there is hope for him.

I will tell you how you can begin changing your child's diet for the better; how to track down some of his hidden food allergies, food sensitivities, and other conditions that might be causing him to have behavioral and/or learning problems. I will explain the problems associated with the hyperactive child and describe some practical ways to deal with them.

Your child's future depends entirely on you. The love and help you give him when he needs you the most will stay with him the rest of his life. As you guide him down the road to health and happiness, you can help him function well both mentally and physically.

This book is meant to be a guideline for bewildered parents of a problem child. It is based on experience and research. I have become a believer in good nutrition and a natural and allergy-free diet, because I have learned first-hand how beneficial they were to my own child.

This is also the story of my exceptional son, Harris, his struggle to cope with hyperkinesis, and his infinite courage, despite his small stature, which led to success.

Janey Walls Mitchell

A mother's tears flow freely when her child is handicapped physically, mentally, or emotionally, or with a complex combination of problems. Because of the child, she sheds tears of frustration, hope, disappointment, relief, hopelessness, joy and anger. But most of all, she sheds tears of love.

God knows her plight. She prays for an answer . . .

# PART I
## Our Ultimate Triumph

# 1. The Bubble Burst

I stood in stunned silence, staring at what was left of the bicycle Harris had wrecked in his rage. He had stripped out the bolts, thrown away the parts, bent the spokes and let the air out of the tires. He had then taken a can of purple paint to the ugly shambles. All this because his dad had refused to let him play video games until his poor grades improved.

This was not the first time Harris's bicycle was his rampage victim, but it was the last. It was also a turning point in our lives.

The previous week, for some unknown reason, Harris had become upset with the whole family and flushed all our toothbrushes down the toilet. Seething with anger, we dished out thirty dollars for the plumber's fee, and vowed to make him a different child. Now he had destroyed his bicycle, and we had to act on that vow. But how?

Like most parents with this problem, we got a heap of advice on how to raise our frenetic child. But we had already tried most of it. He still remained a constant problem.

Spanking had little effect. Pain of any kind didn't seem to faze him. In fact, he usually struck out at us, clawing, kicking and screaming, with senseless speech spewing from his fiery red face. Afterward, he would swear incoherently. To contain him was impossible. During one of his tantrums, he was almost stronger than we were. We usually ended up as the victims.

We had tried every disciplinary approach with no success. Privileges were withdrawn: no television, no talking on the phone, no visiting at friends' homes, earlier bedtime, stints in the corner, added chores—the same things most parents do for punishment. Nothing worked.

Harris is a handsome, curly-haired blond, with sensitive blue eyes. Freckles are splashed across his pudgy nose. He will soon be entering high school — a changed person from four years ago.

This is what our thin-as-a-rail son used to be like: part imp, part angel. He used to talk a mile a minute. He was a boisterous bundle of energy, a perpetual motion machine, and a perplexing paradox in personality. He could be soft, cheerful, charming, and a sheer joy, then in his role reversal, a mad lion out of its cage. He possessed a warm sense of humor, often erupting with unexpected quips.

Even before he burst from my womb, he was a real livewire. At birth, we realized we had no ordinary child. As he grew and matured, his uncontrollable temper tantrums grew worse and more frequent. They became a daily occurrence. He would often lie on the floor screaming at the top of his lungs, kicking with all his might. Afterward, he was exhausted and irritable.

Life was a see-saw experience, going through bad and good cycles. Although at times, he had many stimulating qualities, he often was dreadful. He did everything opposite to what we taught him to do, though often involuntarily.

Like a simmering volcano, he had spasmodic eruptions. His daily outbursts had a negative effect on our lives. Yet I felt there was little to be done in the way of controlling him. I didn't seek outside help until his problems became too severe to endure, because I felt there was none.

Harris's sparkling blue eyes, winsome smile and his sometimes warm personality made the pitfalls more tolerable. Prayer sustained me, but I was weak and worn.

One moment I wanted desperately to hug and kiss him and pretend he was a trouble-free child — like the time he asked, "Mother, when is Jesus coming down here? I hope it's before I grow up."

The next minute he would bug me to utter exasperation! He would respond, "Yes, sir!" instead of the proper "Yes, ma'am." Or again, when I called "Harris!" he would respond, "That's my name, don't wear it out!" Nothing short of a severe lashing could make him change his stubborn tune.

Harris, eight years old at this point, was living in a bizarre Jekyll-Hyde body, never knowing what it would do from one minute to the next. My heart wept for him. I prayed for a key to unlock the door to his emotional prison.

I was a desperate mother searching for a solution to a perplexing problem which had become unbearable. Harris was hyperactive. It was almost more than I could stand. My life seemed constantly to be turned upside down and nothing ever seemed to be in order.

Like other parents in the same situation, I wondered how this could happen to me. I knew Harris was not like a "normal" child. When I dreamed of becoming a parent, I imagined I would have a perfectly "normal" child, with the same problems and pleasures other children have. Instead, his problems were unimaginable and his pleasures few.

Before his birth, my own life experiences were hardly ever what I had visualized, but I could handle most of the problems that drifted my way. Then I had this child who failed to meet any of my expectations whatsoever. The troubles each day were such that they drained me of all my strength — mentally, physically, and emotionally.

A mother feels tremendous guilt when she admits to herself that she is disappointed in the kind of child she has conceived. These feelings only add to the misery caused by his behavior. We all suffer emotionally when we have to give up idealistic dreams for almost unbearable reality.

Our other child — tall, lanky, good-natured, brown-haired Steven, has always been much different. Four years older than Harris, he talks with his incredibly blue eyes. They dance with good humor as he jokes, and laughter fills the air around him. We never hear any complaints about him, only compliments.

During the summer months, he used to stay with my parents, who live two thousand miles away. My mother summed Steven up best:

"He's mannerly and well-behaved. He's happy-go lucky and spreads sunshine wherever he goes. He has a smile on his face when he goes to bed and a smile on his face when he wakes up. You can't ask anymore from a child than that."

But Harris was the terror of the neighborhood. He seemed to bring trouble to all. I grieved to see him so lonely and disliked. He would make many friends — and lose them the same day. I grew tired of all the complaints I heard about him, because I knew only too well how true they were.

My heart silently cried for him — like the time when he and two best friends had played together all day. The two friends were going to spend the night together. Harris, on the other hand, was being sent home because one of the boys' mothers proclaimed, "Harris is a pain! I can't stand him!" Harris came home sobbing.

Or like the time when I got a phone call saying he was kicked out of Cub Scouts — the weekly activity he always looked forward to — because his disruptive behavior disturbed the other children. When told of his fate, his face became pale, his eyes wide and horror-stricken.

"Mom, I really try to be good there. You know how much I love it! When the other kids pick on me, I just go tell the teacher, but she won't do anything about it. She seems to think it's always my fault."

He then walked slowly into his room, shut the door, laid down on his bed and cried uncontrollably.

I was paralyzed by guilt and plagued with inner recriminations. Was I somehow to blame for Harris's condition? I thought of myself as worthless, nothing more than a total failure. Where had I failed? I wallowed in self-pity.

"Why me, Lord?" I questioned.

I was ashamed and embarrassed because of Harris's behavior before friends, relatives and strangers. What must they think of me as a mother? Many times I wished the same thing could happen to me that usually happens in a James Bond scene — that the floor underneath would just give way and I could disappear from view!

Other people often acted negatively toward Harris, which would put me on the defensive. He was a child who was impossible to enjoy, and I was reminded of this fact daily.

But there were times when my joy and love for him would run high. For instance, when I answered his questions, he would sing out cheerfully "Thought so!" whether or not he knew the answer.

When he was happy he referred to me in his own little nickname, "Moomhead." When he was in an especially good mood, he would singsong, "Moomhead, I love you," or "You're the wonderfulest mother in the world!" The trouble dimmed and I would be caught in the grip of his warmth and charm.

Each family member was affected by Harris's presence. Every home where there is a hyperactive child follows the same pattern — a quarrelsome atmosphere, filled with tension. Hyperactivity can cause emotional problems in the family as well as the child.

My husband, Beau, and I bickered over our child. We could never agree on our disciplinary approaches. I felt he was too strict. He felt I was over-protective. Our quarrels usually exploded with:

"You're too strict! You're like a drill sergeant! You nag, scream and criticize him too much!"

"You're not strict enough! You mother him too much. You do everything for him!"

Then Harris would break in with, "Are you two going to get a divorce? It's all my fault!"

Harris often wished he had never been born, because he caused so much havoc. He felt our household would be much happier without him.

Beau is a hyperactive blue-eyed blond. His temperament is similar to Harris's. Since hyperactivity is often hereditary, I began to harbor resentment that Beau was to blame for our son's problems. As if he had done it purposely!

Beau had been chronically tense, irritable, and short-tempered. In his thirties we learned, by accident, that Beau is hyperactive. When he asked the doctor for some diet pills to help him lose a few pounds, the doctor gave him the amphetamine-type drug, Eskatrol. It changed his disposition. His fits of temper no longer were an hourly occurrence. He was quieter, no longer talking full-speed like a 78 rpm record being played at 33⅓ rpm. He was pleasant to be around. He was calm.

Beau noticed most his increased attention span. He was able to concentrate fully, to think more clearly, and to remain patient for long periods of time. When he was on Eskatrol, he was a changed person. (We were to learn later from Harris's doctor that stimulants have a reverse effect and act as "downers" in hyperactive children.)

Our home has seen its share of arguments, slammed doors, hurt feelings — and apologies. Our opposing viewpoints were not always discussed rationally. But when we finally stopped orchestrating blame, we began to restructure our own behavior to become more effective parents.

It was an overwhelming ordeal for me to be a parent of a hyperactive child. I had no prior experience, but I knew he needed love and acceptance. My ultimate goal was to make Harris feel loved, wanted and accepted in spite of the trouble he caused. At the time, however, I didn't realize that diet could help me achieve this goal as well as make him a calm, likeable person. Like most parents, we responded automatically to the echoes of "Let's go to McDonald's!"

Saying, "I love Harris" sounds so simple. But loving him meant helping him and giving of myself. When Harris didn't measure up to what I had expected, I felt disappointed and gypped. I was full of self-blame. I felt I had failed as a parent, and therefore was unworthy of life's pleasures. I had a sense of missing out.

It was difficult for me to be satisfied with what I had. I improved my situation, however, by bringing my goals and ambitions into focus, making them reasonable and achievable. I acknowledged that the most rewarding accomplishments in life were those for which we paid more dearly.

Once I stopped my self-recrimination, it was easier to help Harris cope. I worked in a positive direction to give him loving care and guidance by discovering techniques — which I will describe to you —which brought us good results.

When he was six, I began taking Harris to various doctors. I found I had to prove he was hyperactive. I listed his schoolteacher and the school nurse, along with many friends, neighbors and grocery clerks, for the doctor to talk with, who would confirm my case. It's no mystery when a child has this affliction. Everyone is aware of it!

The best proof I had, however, was when Harris sat in the doctor's office for a half hour. He began his usual mistreatment of the magazines, rolling them around on the floor, screaming, talking loudly, crying, and bothering other children. Soon everyone in the waiting room was staring.

The examining room was no different. While we waited, Harris's hands were busily trying to play with the blood pressure gauge, cotton tips, and other paraphernalia. It was impossible to keep him still.

The doctor remarked that — although it was not the case with Harris — sometimes a hyperactive child might appear perfectly normal on a one-to-one basis, such as in a doctor's office, but not in a schoolroom with thirty other children. He said there are too many distractions, such as sights, sounds, things, children to touch, etc.

We left with the confirmed diagnosis of hyperkinesis, along with a prescription for a drug: Dexedrine. Dexedrine is a stimulant, but surprisingly, the doctor said that stimulants have a reverse effect and act as "downers" in hyperactive children. This was the first of a series of drugs prescribed for Harris's disorder. The others were Deaner, Ritalin, and Cylert. Each had a similar effect and worked quite well, except for the many side-effects. Each time I ceased using the drug, grasping for a miracle as we roamed from doctor to doctor. But each new doctor only prescribed a different drug.

I was skeptical. I had reservations.

Were drugs the only answer? My instincts said they were not. Drugs were merely covering up his problem, not eliminating the cause. They did help Harris, though, by calming him down, stretching his attention span and allowing him to cope with his environment.

I thought of friends who had taken their hyperactive child to the family doctor. He suggested tranquilizers — for the parents, not the child! Today this child is institutionalized. I didn't want this for Harris!

When Harris was barely ten years old — the day he wrecked his bicycle — I came to the end of my rope. I knew I had to stop looking for people and things to blame and start looking for solutions. I knew something had to be done to make Harris better. I also knew that whatever happened had to be an improvement. He could not have grown any worse. I could not live this way forever, trying to deal with his Jekyll-Hyde personality. I didn't want him to become a juvenile delinquent. I felt in my heart there were many good possibilities for him.

If I could only program myself to have the necessary energy, enthusiasm and ambition, then I could achieve. No longer would I stagnate, expecting my troubles to magically disappear. I vowed to put forth a special effort to solve my problems. I had to plunge full-speed ahead with determination and dedication — the root of every successful undertaking.

I was fortunate enough then to find a doctor with a hyperactive child of his own. He was the one person who understood. He strongly believed that diet affects behavior. He helped pave the way to success through natural food and an allergy-free diet.

At this point, I began to take a personal interest in nutrition. I read every book, magazine, medical journal — all I could find on the subject. I found and soaked up a wealth of information. I searched for books, trying to learn more about the hyperkinetic syndrome. I picked the brains of specialists who were kind and generous to share their time and expertise, and I talked with parents of children with similar ailments.

This was a turning point in my life. Before long, I was a wiser person. I had a burning desire to continue searching and experimenting. I emerged inspired and enlightened, because I had reached out for answers. But I didn't accept any pat answers. I listened, researched, questioned, evaluated and trusted my own judgment on my way toward achieving my goal.

I had faith that I could find some way to solve all the problems. We could then live a more enjoyable life. I began working industriously toward helping Harris have some calmness and control in his life through changing his diet. We worked together as a team, believing that we would find favorable results.

It seems unfair at times that we are not all blessed with an equal amount of hardships or joys in our lives! But life isn't meant to be that way. I realized I had to accept my plight and do my best. I had the choice of changing the situation, or learning to adjust to it the way it was. I opted for change.

I responded to something negative within my life and made something positive out of it. I looked at our obstacles as challenges and turned the challenges into accomplishments. Harris is a unique individual who had the direction of his life changed.

We live in a society of fast foods, instant replays on TV, computers, charge cards, automatic household helpers, world-wide telephone communications and men walking on the moon. An aspirin makes a headache disappear and Penicillin cures pneumonia. Why won't Ritalin or Cylert cure hyperactivity?

I did not find easy answers or simple cures, but I did find answers. I also found that love and wishful thinking are not enough.

## 2. Child Renewal

Several months had passed since the bicycle incident. It was a cool, misty fall day as I sat in our car watching Harris traipse from house to house trying to sell magazine subscriptions. He asked each person, "Would you like to buy a magazine subscription? They're really a good bargain. It's so we can raise money for our class trip to Sacramento."

The answer from nearly every person was "No." Others merely slammed the door in his face.

Harris had worked diligently trying to sell the subscriptions. Everyone else in his classroom had sold at least one. This meant that each child had a "mag-man weepul" — a little furry button — tagged on his or her shirt. This button was the prize for selling the first subscription. In essence, the mag-man weepul signified success.

For the tenth sale, a child received a mag-man blinking visor. I wasn't exactly sure what this visor was, but to watch Harris describe it as his eyes grew saucer-big, I could tell that it was the ultimate prize.

What was so different about the way Harris repeatedly encountered rejection was his reaction. He was remaining calm. He didn't spiral into a state of agitated explosiveness, stomp his feet, throw his hands up in the air and declare, "The dumb people won't buy any! They're all stupid! I'm quitting!" Instead he stuck with it unruffled, and accepted rejection.

Although anger didn't overtake him, tears eventually did well within. He finally said, "Mom, people just aren't buying today. Maybe we can come back tomorrow, if it's okay with you."

And that we did.

I knew the instant I saw his face the next day what the outcome had been. His feet bounced, tousling his golden hair. His cheeks were flushed with excitement and his teeth were flashing a broad smile.

"Mom! I sold one! The lady in the green house bought it! She even thanked me for coming by!"

His spirits were soaring. He would finally get to own a mag-man weepul!

"Mom, can we come back tomorrow so I can sell nine more?" he pleaded. "Then I can get a mag-man hat that blinks pretty lights."

Sure enough, he sold the remaining nine by the end of the week.

Monday afternoon, I was at the window waiting for him to come home from school. I spied flashing red, green, and yellow lights on a green visor. Harris's face was the picture of happiness as he proudly modeled the hat, a symbol of a long-awaited accomplishment.

Harris has made a tremendous transition. He is a totally different child. Diet therapy has brought many favorable changes in our lives. Diet *can* change a child's behavior, attitude . . . and life.

The new Harris is a joy to the entire family. He is everything we had hoped for in a son.

Harris wakes up rejuvenated, eager to meet the challenge of another day.

His self-esteem is shooting uphill. He likes himself, and cares about other people.

He finally enjoys school, refusing to miss unless absolutely necessary. The last time I made a dental appointment for him during school hours, he cried and pleaded with me to change it.

He is doing much better with his schoolwork and isn't restless or easily distracted. His attention span has stretched. His last quarterly progress report reflected the improvement.

Harris rushed eagerly into the kitchen, delightedly smiling from ear to ear. He thumped the report down on the table.

"Looky there!" he chuckled.

All six of his junior high school teachers had filled it out. On all except the last one, was written "Harris is doing fine," "Good," "Passing" and "Continued good work!"

The last of the six teachers had written in bold letters — "Harris is putting forth much more effort this year. His written work has greatly improved."

Another example of Harris's changed life: he has become our town's "computer whiz kid." He swiftly caught on to the computer's complex functions, because of his new ability to concentrate.

The news of his computer ability quickly got around.

Our personal finances wouldn't allow purchase of a computer, but a nearby dealer had one on display. Harris used it daily. He sat for hours at a time playing and creating different programs. It was intriguing to watch his small fingers dance over the keys.

I called the store manager to make sure it was all right if Harris stayed there for such long periods of time. I didn't want him to become a nuisance. The manager surprised me by saying that Harris was so exceptional on the machine that he was helping sell computers!

The manager refused to let other children use them. He said Harris knew the computers better than anyone else, and that he was the only child who behaved well!

The following year, when Harris took computers as an elective in school, he topped the class. He often had to show the instructor how to figure out the computer!

Harris has many friends now. There are no more fights. Recently, he missed being elected class representative by one class vote. He didn't vote for himself! Nonetheless, he was bubbling over for having so many friends.

Harris has learned to handle some of the stresses in his life. He no longer bites his fingernails.

Like any other child, he still has some bad habits — he still answers me "Yes, sir!" and his fingerprints still are embedded above each doorway — but even children who aren't hyperactive leave plenty of those. I am not pretending he is flawless. His life is far from perfect, but it is far better than it was a few years ago.

Many of our friends and relatives now are firm believers in a comprehensive treatment for the hyperactive child, no longer believing it was just another phase or "fad" of mine. Many labeled me as a nutritional "freak," but now they know it works.

It is better to show by example rather than by preaching. It was exciting and touching to watch Harris improve. I had seen him suffering so much! I asked him now how he felt.

He thought and answered softly, "My body is calm."

What success! You, too, can find the same kind of success. It takes determination, patience, and willingness to work, but it is a fabulous feeling when a child becomes a bona fide delight.

Although Harris no longer wrecks his bicycle, he does know how to take it apart, repair it, and put every piece back properly. Due to his former temper, our teenager is a good bicycle mechanic. In fact, a gold trophy adorns his dresser as a first-place prize in bicycle racing, and a new Mongoose frame — his cherished dream — is on his bike. A front-page newspaper picture of his racing achievement decorates his wall.

Harris taught me how much I truly loved him. His bad conduct motivated me to find a solution to his hyperactivity. I am proud of Harris. Without his cooperation and diligence, it would never have been possible. He followed through on everything I learned, although not all efforts were successful.

I know I have instilled a belief in good nutrition that will stay with him. He will keep his behavior within acceptable bounds in spite of his hyperkinetic syndrome. The signs will always be lurking in the shadows of his life, but he will be in control. Harris will always have to control his diet, but at least he knows exactly what he can or cannot eat.

I really appreciate how far he has come, because he has worked so much harder for his progress than the average child. He knows he must work hard to win, but he knows he can win.

I once dreaded the future. Not anymore.

I have many dreams I hope Harris will fulfill, but I am realistic in my expectations. I know he is not capable of perfection. If he has a good self-image and does something worthwhile and satisfying to him ... that's what counts.

I am grateful to the growing body of physicians and specialists now exploring the causes and treatment of hyperactivity. It is comforting to have support when we face frustration, despair, exhaustion, and criticism.

I am also grateful to the many unforgettable parents who have been gracious enough to share their encounters.

My greatest gratitude goes to God, who showered me with His love. He gave me guidance and was there when I needed him, which was often. Through my darkest hours, highest moments and ultimate triumph, I was aware of His presence.

My hope is that some day hyperactivity and its causes may be recognized with dignity and authority, and the treatment followed courageously.

A six-year-old neighbor boy made Beau realize what I was trying to accomplish with Harris.

Beau told the boy I was a "health nut."

"Do you know what a health nut is?" he questioned the lad.

"Sure," was the reply. "It's someone who cares about their health."

All aspects of my life have changed since Harris's diet transition. We are a much happier and more contented family. Our lives are more complete. Our home is filled with love and better understanding. Our story has a more-than-happy ending.

Harris used to tease, "I climbed Mt. Everest!" In a sense he has. He had a lot of hard falls on the way, but he kept climbing. We all have won the battle.

Thomas Fuller sums up my feelings best. "Happy is he who is happy in his children."

You, too, can find our kind of happiness. Hope lies ahead.

# PART II
# On the Road to Success

# 3. Sweep Away Guilt

Guilt — that gnawing feeling haunts the parents of a hyperactive child. Guilty feelings are an everyday occurrence. They can keep us from being effective parents and properly functioning human beings.

I have talked with many parents of hyperactive children who feel this way. They blame themselves for the problem and believe they may have done something wrong to cause it.

These parents feel inadequate and worthless, just as I did. They feel that they have failed as parents. They don't know how to help their child and have grown tired of outlandish conduct and demands. They are in despair, and can see only more trouble ahead.

To make matters worse, others are ready to reinforce those guilty feelings. They remark that the child is spoiled, neglected, or needs punishment. They imply that the parents need lessons on how to raise children!

No wonder we feel worthless, rejected and guilty! It is natural for us to blame ourselves when other parents we know don't have these problems.

It is only natural to be angry and discouraged with a problem child. But these guilt feelings only make us look for something or someone to blame, instead of looking for solutions.

It is important to recognize that we did not cause the problem and that we can do something about it. Parents need to be reassured that *inadequate parenting did not make the child hyperactive!* The following story of Duane, "normal" brother of a hyperactive boy, is a case in point.

When Duane was two, his divorced mother married Duane's stepdad, who was severely hyperactive. They eventually had a hyperactive son, Kevin, who was just like his dad. Kevin was ill-tempered and a troublemaker, fighting constantly with other children. He was rude, selfish, friendless and a poor student. Kevin's parents heard constant complaints from his teachers. At age ten, Kevin was given the drug Cylert, which helped him function more effectively.

On the opposite side, Duane, at thirteen, was a warm, kind, unselfish, even-tempered, good-hearted human being. He made friends easily, did well in school and obeyed his parents.

Duane and Kevin were raised in the same home. Did inadequate parenting make the one child hyperactive? *No!*

## Parenting is a Tough Job

It takes all of our resources to raise a normal child. No other time in history have we had so much to watch for in our children's growth and development — and so little time in which to do it.

Nothing in life prepares parents to bring up a problem child. Friends, relatives, doctors, and sometimes strangers are ready to offer advice. But have they raised a child like this one? Do they really know how he can keep a home in disorganized turmoil?

Most people don't realize emotional problems can be a tremendous handicap. They think of a handicap as being physical. There is a world of difference between *knowing* a hyperactive child and *living* with one.

The hyperactive child's erratic behavior affects everyone in the family, even the pets. As a result, the strain often becomes unbearable. Feelings of hopelessness and inadequacy can push the parents into deep depression. In fact, it is hard to hide dissatisfaction with the child.

It is important to realize, however, that *the emotional problems within the home have been caused by the presence of hyperactivity. It does not mean that the emotional problems caused the hyperactivity.*

It is important to talk about our feelings with other parents in the same boat. We can support one another through understanding. It is also good to glean ideas from other parents. When we hear advice from those with the same problems, we can trust it. This advice carries more weight. We can take it seriously and act on it.

## Negative Sensations

We parents sometimes find it hard to respond to the child in a positive way. We want to love him, yet he seems to fail us at every turn. We always hope tomorrow will be different, yet wake up to find it is not.

We will promise ourselves not to scream or spank, and not to get upset with his naughtiness and demands. We will promise ourselves "never again" after losing our temper, but it will happen again. We are human. We may make a bad situation worse by constant worry and the feeling that we are trapped.

Many parents are being truthful when they say they have tried everything and nothing works. They have probably tried every imaginable disciplinary approach with little success. Sometimes they allow the child to do as he wishes to relieve the pressure. This places a strain on the entire family. Each parent will blame the other for actions that caused the problem.

There are many times when parents feel they cannot face another day with their impossible, crabby, disgruntled child and his "revved up" motor. They cannot accept their child. Their feelings are akin to hate for the continual disruption.

All such parents of hyperactive children have these frightening feelings. That's why we feel guilty. We wouldn't be human if we never experienced such feelings.

Some parents strike out in anger, then feel hate and disgust toward themselves. Others turn to alcohol or drugs. The problems are a constant reminder of hopelessness.

Remember, all parents say and do things they regret. We should not berate ourselves for the mistakes we have made in the past. Most parents fight over how their children should be raised. We must not let our emotions hold us back from being effective parents.

Bill and Joyce disagreed on how their eight-year-old son, Ross, should be handled. They were pulling in opposite directions. Bill felt Ross needed stern discipline, while Joyce let Ross have his own way. Their marriage began to crumble. They eventually sought counseling for themselves and their son.

## Job Training

Just because we are parents does not guarantee us adequate parenting skills. Most parents have trouble raising their children because they have not been trained to be a parent. Training is acquired through experience, but everyone is an amateur when it comes to raising children. We learn how to handle one child and the next child will be altogether different.

Parents must have confidence in themselves. This will lead the child to have a favorable self-image. The more confident we are, the more assured the child will be. When we are not self-assured, it is best not to show it.

Parents who devalue themselves through lack of confidence become resentful and critical of the child. When parents are able to control hyperactivity, they gain more confidence, and the child benefits.

We need to accept ourselves as we are, then we can rebuild our lives and positive feelings. For example: One particularly bad day, I broke into tears, full of self-pity.

Harris wrapped his scrawny arms around me and said, "I love you, Moomhead."

Suddenly my mind glided into another world. His caring made my problems less overwhelming. These loving feelings helped strengthen the bond between us. When Harris has a sunny smile and good disposition, there is sunshine all around.

Regardless of how we try, we cannot change a child's temperament. However, we can provide an atmosphere that will promote a good self-image and help him not to feel inferior. We can help him reach his potential, in spite of his hyperactivity. By nurturing a positive attitude, we can neutralize many forces working against him.

We need to "turn the negative into the positive." It is important to set the goals in accordance with the child's strengths and weaknesses. Sometimes failures and disappointments are blessings in disguise, allowing us to reassess our goals.

The hyperactive child can change the direction of his life. One of his greatest strengths will be the conviction that he has the power to grow and mature, conquer his environment and "make it" in his journey through life. When he has confidence in himself, obstacles can turn into challenges and challenges into accomplishments.

Poor work records lead to unhappiness. We must accept the fact that we cannot change all things. We need to accept what we cannot change and confront head-on those things we can. We must stop focusing on what is missing in the child's life and seek what is there.

Each family situation has its own unique set of characteristics. No parent or home is perfect. That is reality!

There is no recipe measuring discipline, education, patience, understanding, tears, and love for the production of a model child. We do the best job we can, but guilt still lurks over our shoulders. Just don't give in to it!

# 4. From Rock Bottom

Scott, a handsome, blond eight-year-old with ocean-blue eyes, pushed his best friend's bicycle down a steep embankment, laughing all the while. He turned on his buddy and began punching him repeatedly, as other bewildered children watched.

The abused friend wiped the blood from his nose and cried, "Why did ya do that for?"

Scott replied, "I dunno! I just wanted to."

Only two days earlier Scott had gone to a neighbor's home to watch some young people swim and play badminton. Scott stole money from several wallets in the dressing room. He was caught, but denied the misdeed and shamelessly claimed the money was saved from his allowance.

These were typical occurrences in Scott's life. His mother, Shirley, said his last three years had been marked by constant restless activity, refusal to cooperate with parents and teachers, failing grades, frequent fights with other children, stealing, lying, fire-starting, sneaking out nights — the list goes on and on.

Scott is a typical hyperactive child.

Inevitably, Shirley came to the end of her rope, as I did, and vowed to "do something!"

"I could no longer endure it," she said. "Life seemed unbearable. Scott's problems were multiplying."

Thanks to a new lifestyle, Scott made a radical change in behavior. He now is nice to have around. His constant fights have stopped. He is doing remarkably well in school, and again he is welcome in neighbors' yards. Shirley says he feels good about himself, not confused, unhappy or unsuccessful.

How did this mother bring about such a radical change in the life of her hyperactive child?

Through diet.

Specialists, physicians and some parents have been promoting the idea that poor diet and/or food allergies, food sensitivities and food additives can cause a wide range of behavioral and physical problems in some individuals. These parents have come to realize that what their children eat has very much to do with their behavioral patterns, as well as their mental and physical development.

No specialist claims to have all the answers to every problem of the hyperactive child, but they do believe sincerely that many children can be helped by changing their diet. Furthermore, they believe that even non-problem children can benefit from a better diet.

Many parents, like Shirley, are witnessing dramatic changes in their children and breathing sighs of relief. They are firm believers that diet has a lot to do with changed attitudes and behavior. Many have also found that they are able to reduce or eliminate medication for hyperactivity by changing their children's diet.

Hyperactivity has grown from a rarely discussed disorder to a household word. Since the number of afflicted children has increased, and since successful research has gone on, doctors and parents are becoming more familiar and better informed about the syndrome.

Parents are realizing that their children's overall well-being cannot be left only to doctors. A good share of the responsibility falls on their shoulders, and they are taking an active part in helping the body to heal itself.

It is extremely difficult to change a hyperactive child into a normal, healthy, productive, self-controlled adult. There are many steps, however, that parents can take to help their child. The sooner they start, the better.

## The Gist of the Situation

It seemed like every doctor (and there were many) kept repeating, "He'll outgrow it," or "Learn to live with it." I knew this was not always first-rate advice. Sometimes we have to follow our hearts and take matters into our own hands.

I knew that children might not "outgrow" it; that they could become hyperactive adults, with tendencies toward depression, suicide, guilt, distrust, anger, alcoholism and other negative emotions. I knew Harris might suffer the rest of his life, and so I decided I would help him cope with it now.

According to a study in 1974 by Maurice Bowerman, seventy-five percent of today's prisoners were hyperactive children.[1] This study scared the wits out of me.

Beware of the statement, "He'll outgrow it." It encourages parents to do nothing, thinking he will. Help your child. Even a little improvement is better than none. If you do nothing now, you will regret it later.

Ann, a divorcee and the mother of Terry, a sixteen-year-old hyperactive, can vouch for this. She says her son is a bum. He steals, gets mad and breaks up the furniture, curses, and hits her. She is often beside herself with anxiety and fear. She tries everything to please Terry, but nothing works.

Terry is a school dropout. He could never conform. He often comes home intoxicated, but denies drinking.

"If only I had got help for Terry in his younger years," Ann moans. "At sixteen, it may be too late."

Terry was picked up by the police for burglary and is presently in jail.

Many are trained to help hyperactive children — in nutrition, medicine, psychology, education, and counseling. It is important, however, that they be consulted early, not when it's too late. Parents cannot wait until he "grows out of it." Chances are, he will not. The effort needs to be made now. Parents can help prevent years of sorrow and anguish for themselves and their child by acting early.

It is often a parent, usually the mother, who recognizes that the child needs help. Frequently, fathers seem not to realize that anything much is wrong. Sometimes a father hates to admit that his child (especially a son) is different, not the normal child. At times, one parent has to take responsibility when he or she realizes something is wrong, because it is vital to get help.

Most books on hyperactivity discuss how to control a child with anything from coffee to rewards for good behavior; from drugs to psychiatric help to psychosurgery. They usually say nothing about food additives, food allergies, food sensitivities or numerous other problems caused by a poor diet. If we can rid the child of these, he can probably improve because he wants to, not because he has to.

I am convinced, after thorough reading and study (now here comes this book's bombshell, which I will back up with evidence) that *food allergy and a sensitivity to sugar are major causes of hyperactivity.*

## We Sow and Reap

Every parent's hope is for his or her child to learn how to control his behavior to be acceptable to others, to realize his maximum potential, and to be otherwise well-adjusted. Armed with the information in this book, this goal can be achieved, even by the parents of a hyperactive child.

Although a hyperactive child is severely handicapped by his symptoms, once he is on the pathway to control, he will be able to contain himself. His handicap can be turned into "handicapable."

Parents can give the creative incentive their child needs to fill his reservoirs with positives for a fulfilling and rewarding existence. Thinking in positive terms, he can become an accepted individual, with good and bad points. Then he can be helped to have control of his life for a future of confidence and optimism. His life can be changed drastically, as my son's was, through diet change. Diet does affect behavior.

I cannot promise an easy solution. There is no magic cure-all for hyperactivity. But your child can be controlled or, at least, improved. It will take detective work on your part, but you have nothing to lose but time, and you have everything to gain.

It will take patience, understanding, and love. But someday you can take your child into a food store and know he won't tear the food off the shelves or lie down and scream his head off. You will find he no longer creates chaos routinely. You will be able to be proud of him. And as his hyperactivity and its associated problems decrease, you will find your own physical and emotional strains are relieved.

We need to proceed optimistically, showing our children we love and want to care for them. This not only is the first day of the rest of our lives, but of our children's, as well. We need to make it count!

Take Susan, the mother of six-year-old hyperactive Darrell, as an example. When she had an inkling that diet might control Darrell's hyperactivity, instead of taking an "I'll give it a try and see what happens" attitude, she was optimistic. She said, "I know Darrell will improve." She set her goal, believing in a successful outcome, and worked toward it. Susan's total faith and enthusiasm worked. Darrell's rapid behavioral transition was astounding.

## Trial and Error

Results of a diet change can be remarkably rewarding and well worth the effort. The entire family's life can change for the better, but it takes trial and error, with faith thrown in. Although there is no guarantee that it will work for every child, it is worth an all-out effort for everyone's sake. The child will learn to like himself and others. He will become a positive force in society instead of a menace.

Beau and I spent huge sums taking Harris to various specialists, several out of state, unsuccessfully trying to find a medical solution to his problems. It wasn't until I decided to take action myself that I finally found the answer. I simply couldn't bear our chaotic lifestyle any longer. I was ready and willing to try anything.

Many parents will find themselves in the same boat. They try everything and go everywhere in a desperate search for help. Many times they know the direction in which they are headed, but don't know which way to turn.

The comfort and peace we have found has made all the trouble more than worthwhile. I will always be willing to stick to the program, no matter how troublesome. Our well-being is ample reward.

I know from personal experience that the effort to maintain the diet is a monumental task, but the child's future is at stake. Ask yourself how much time, energy and money have you already spent repairing the damage done by your child. Like me, you probably try to keep one step ahead of him, without much success. I can't count the times I wished I could vanish into thin air over the embarrassment Harris caused me. I decided to stop suffering when I saw a way out.

The child can and should be helped without using drugs, but at times, even drugs might be necessary. Many specialists recommend drugs only until the nutritional approach has had time to take effect (typically three to four weeks).

There is increased recognition among specialists, physicians, nutritionists, teachers, and parents of hyperactive and/or learning-disabled children that nutritional elements do play an essential role in how a child feels, acts and functions.

## Stop the Merry-Go-Round

As you begin to understand how your child functions biochemically, you can change his eating habits to calm him down and allow him to develop social skills. If he is one of the fortunate ones, you will see improvement in about two weeks, maybe sooner. But some children take as long as six weeks. Be patient!

Harris was on the diet only two days before I noticed a remarkable improvement in his behavior.

Since no two hyperactive children share exactly the same symptoms or causes, I cannot guarantee instant results. But you will not regret starting on the road to peace and serenity. If improvement isn't as speedy as you think it should be, don't panic or give up. Each case varies.

It serves as more of an incentive for the child if the whole family adheres to the diet. They may all show improvement, too. If your child's problems are caused by a relatively non-nutritional diet, low blood sugar (worse before meals, better after meals), food allergies, or food sensitivities, he may have inherited it. Other family members may have the very same food-related problems and will benefit from a better diet.

If others have been plagued by fatigue, irritability, depression, headaches, susceptibility to infection, or other psychosomatic complaints, the diet may make them disappear. It is an indescribably good feeling when the whole family's nerves settle down.

Any diet requires a period of adjustment for the whole family, but you can look forward to a better, more promising tomorrow. We know that without change, life can be nothing short of miserable for all concerned.

Martha, mother of a hyperactive child, says that changing her child's diet has had an effect on the lifestyle of all the family. "Our frequent illnesses, restlessness and grumpiness disappeared," she observed.

## Never Say Quit

The first few weeks of the diet were the hardest for me. It was time-consuming, confusing, restrictive, and frustrating. When I saw the list of forbidden foods, I was overwhelmed, but decided to give it my best. It was worth it!

Extra time was required for grocery shopping, menu planning and meal preparation until I finally got the hang of it. Then it went like a whiz. And soon I found that it took far less time to adhere strictly to the diet than it had required to manage Harris through a typical day before we went on the diet.

I became discouraged many times while trying to solve my son's severe problems. I felt I wasn't getting anywhere. If your child also is severely hyperactive, there may be slack periods when nothing is accomplished, when you are unable to pinpoint the problem food. Wait it out or go on to something else. Don't give up. And don't become discouraged. Nothing ever runs smoothly, especially when it concerns a hyperactive child. Everything he does is unpredictable. It is not possible for our homes to run smoothly, and it would be foolish for us to hope for it. The important thing to do is hang in there! Be determined to find solutions.

I want you to love, respect, and enjoy your child the way I do mine. You *can* plan your lives together, looking forward to a better controlled, a more enjoyable, satisfying, and rewarding existence. Working together, you can find success. With faith as a motivator, you will win. Faith can move mountains and calm a hyperactive child.

Focus on success rather than failure. Failure is not something we are forced to live with the rest of our lives. As long as we are willing to try to correct our mistakes and learn from them, failures can become successes.

The fact is, you have only satisfaction ahead of you as your child becomes a more manageable child from the tranquilizing effect of an additive-free diet, along with attention to food allergies, food sensitivities, and other things causing his problems.

### New Lease on Life

Even if you succeed with your child as I did with Harris, you will find that all is not rosy. It is never easy to place a child on a specialized diet. Regardless, you will not regret the effort it took to put your child's life in focus. Your spirits will lift when you kiss his terrible tantrums and crankiness goodbye.

Once you make the decision to find control, you will feel confident and peaceful, as I did. Then everything will flow more smoothly. When he makes progress, a burden will be lifted off your shoulders. I know... I've been there.

I don't want you to just love your child. I want you to like your child because a child means just about everything to a parent. I like Harris now, but I couldn't before, although I still loved him. There is a difference!

You, too, can find success by following *The Natural Way Program* which consists of two phases — diet, and vitamin and mineral supplementation.

You are going to be searching like a detective for clues, trying to discover what offending foods "set off" your child. You can expect some blunders and may even find some natural foods to be culprits. But the more you control what the child eats, the greater chance you have of discovering what sets him off. When you peek at the list of forbidden foods and effort involved, don't feel it is an overpowering task. *It's not!* Just consider the rewards of your labor.

If your child is on medication for his hyperactivity, and it is helping, your doctor might be able to reduce or even do away with it. Unlike medication, this diet is harmless and doesn't carry any long-term risks for the child — just good health and good cheer.

## Perseverance Pays

By now I hope you're fired with enthusiasm and determination. Can you hardly wait to get started? Don't expect to wake up tomorrow and find a new child sleeping in his bed. It often takes time. Don't give up in despair when you crash head-on into a new stumbling block. These are often the downfall to many a well-planned venture. So don't declare, "Forget the diet. It's too much trouble!" Stick to it. Don't write off your child as being untreatable without at least giving it a good honest try.

Since your child didn't grow in his condition overnight, it's a sure thing he won't grow out of it overnight. But you can start looking on the brighter side.

This diet cannot and will not succeed without full cooperation from both of you, but you can make a winning team. It will get easier after awhile because you both become more experienced. You can also watch progress being made, and that's encouraging!

This is a journey into a positive nourishment adventure and a calmer life ahead for your child. He will end up finding the world an exciting challenge. You and your child should definitely notice the difference!

# 5. Reinforcement

Trying an elimination diet can be frustrating, especially when you can't seem to get supportive help.

Turn a deaf ear on the non-sympathetic relatives and friends when they say your child should not be deprived of sugar. They, themselves, may be addicted to it. Don't let them tell you it is foolish to think sugar, milk, junk food, or food additives have anything to do with the child's behavior.

Your doctor may think you're wasting your time. Your husband may think you've lost your marbles, and your child may be planning to revolt. Try not to let this dampen your spirits to the point that you wonder if it's really worth it.

I can assure you — *it is!* Take heart! Be firm and assertive!

Perhaps the following illustration of Kim will help give you the encouragement you need: Kim plucked up the courage to place her nine-year-old hyperactive daughter, Marie, on an elimination diet. Marie was wild. Temper tantrums were a daily occurrence. She chattered excessively, was destructive, and had a multitude of school problems. She had been referred to a child psychologist for her emotional problems. She also suffered with a spastic colon.

Kim began diligently jotting down each day in a diet diary what Marie ate so she could identify the most bothersome foods.

Kim faced nothing but negative vibes — first, from her husband, Rob, who himself suffers from the syndrome.

"He's a constant complainer, ill-tempered, tension-fatigued, restless, sickly, always sleepy and can't seem to get his motor going for constructive purposes." Kim said. "He also suffers with low blood sugar and other ailments. In general, he functions poorly in his daily life. He lives on sweets and other junk food and says the health business is a bunch of hogwash!"

Rob was unconvinced that food allergies, food sensitivities, and other substances could have anything to do with how Marie felt and acted.

"After all," he argued, "I'm hyperactive too and I should know!"

Rob offered Kim no supportive help. Instead, he voiced his complaints openly about the steps she was taking.

Kim's mother-in-law took sides with Rob.

Kim's good intentions were met with rejection, rebellion, and much criticism, which she took in stride. The more criticism she got, the more determined she became. She exhibited patience and perseverance in her strong desire to help her child.

"I hid my tears of disappointment and loneliness," Kim said "while I kept on trying to help Marie to be a healthier and happier child."

Kim was near her breaking point when some answers began to surface.

She removed additives and sugar from Marie's diet, then milk and wheat products when her diet diary showed they upset Marie.

"For the first time in Marie's life, she was quiet and subdued," Kim said. "I found her to be sweet, warm, and kind, not at all the horrid child she had been!"

Results of Kim's positive action is testimony to the benefits that can be achieved through love and determination.

It often takes a trial-and-error approach, along with a lot of cooperation from other family members. You don't need a lot of hassling. But even if you're making the effort on your own, with no support, a more nutritious elimination diet certainly can't hurt the child. Besides, what you don't look for, you may not find. So you won't know if certain foods are the culprits for your child's disturbed behavior until you try this method.

It's important to respect the child you want to help and not blame him for his problems. A critical factor in making progress is to have confidence that the child can and will change. It is important to have a positive attitude. It can mean the difference between success or failure.

This is an all-or-nothing program. "Half success" also means "half failure." But even children without the problem can behave and function better with a balanced, nutritional diet, so "whole success" can mean success for the whole family.

In other words, the benefits of sound nutrition are not limited to problem children. Just think . . . if a high-quality diet can restore healthy bodies and minds to problem children, envision the possibilities that can be achieved for optimal health and mental ability in other children!

## Winning the Child

Explain to the child why he has to be on this diet. Ask for his full cooperation, which is a crucial factor. If you can't sell the child, then he won't stick to his diet. His parents can't be in control of his life all the time. Therefore, the largest responsibility for success needs to fall on his shoulders.

A child reacts negatively when he is forced into a new lifestyle. But he will soon adapt to it without much trouble. Harris reacted the way any ordinary child would when he was placed on the diet. He cried. After the initial shock, he was eager to find out why his body wasn't right and how to fix it. As he grew more calm, so did I.

Try to teach your child when he is old enough to read his own body signs (make it a game of discovery) so he can tell you when he is not functioning right. Anything can affect his body. He needs to be on the lookout, as well as his parents. Then, as a team, you can find out why he went haywire and work toward putting him back on the right track. Teamwork can make the difference between success or failure. Ask any football team.

Emphasize the foods your child *can* eat instead of the foods he *can't* eat. If you begin telling him what all he can't eat you will only frighten him. Also, don't tell him right off the bat that this is a lifetime diet. It's a new experience, and it will take time for him to get used to the idea. Wait until he gets over the newness of it and then break the news gently. Harris declared he would stay on the diet until he was forty and not a day longer!

Try to teach your child that there should be absolutely no lunch swapping with his classmates.

Peggy, the mother of seven-year-old Bruce, said, "I spend a half an hour handcrafting his school lunch and he trades it for a cupcake!"

If there are other children within the family, make the ground rules beforehand. Let them know there will be absolutely no teasing concerning the child's diet. Make sure this is clearly understood. Punishment would be in order if the rule is broken. Most children are eager to help their hyperactive sibling cool his explosive temper. They would gladly give six months' allowance to bring some beneficial results. The hyperactive child's success is their success too.

Don't make a habit of continually discussing the diet, but treat it matter-of-factly. The child will soon realize, as Harris did, that the diet makes him feel better.

When the inevitable happens, and your child announces that he is going to abandon his diet, try to stay calm. Don't say that he's going to stick to his diet no matter what. Instead, give him a little "psychological" boost by telling him kindly that you know how difficult it is for him to be so good and stick to his diet.

It's hard for any child to stick to a diet when his friends stop off for candy bars or ice cream. Sympathize with him. Let him know you realize how tough it is. Tell him how strong he is for having done so well. As long as he is trying and is doing the best he can, he needs to be praised.

When the child is honest enough to tell you he has cheated, don't show anger and disappointment. If you do, he won't tell you the next time. Thank him for his honesty. Reassure him, reminding him of the many times he has done well, the progress he is making.

Again, there might be times when he unknowingly eats things he shouldn't, so don't make a big deal of it. Continue to show the child you care and understand when you forbid him to have certain foods so he won't think you're just being mean.

## Road to Regression

When a child is off his diet, he is less reasonable. A vicious cycle develops, because the more he is off his diet, the more he will crave forbidden foods. The more forbidden foods he eats, the more he will want. You can see that when the child goes off his diet a little all the time, it's more difficult for him to stick to it.

Take Eric, for instance: His dad, Martin, insisted they try diet to improve their son's behavior. Although his mother, Sharon, had a sit-back-and-wait-to-see-if-he-grows-out-of-it attitude, she promised she would try the diet to please Martin.

Good results were almost instant. Eric's behavior and grades improved. Then Sharon became more lenient. She began letting Eric have a doughnut here, a candy bar there. Eric began having frequent temper tantrums again. He became testy, unreasonable, and impossible to contend with. He began wanting more sweets than his mother was dishing out. He soon began sneaking them.

He finally announced, "I'm not staying on my diet anymore!"

It is a hardship when other children begin to tease and taunt a child about his diet. It seems that when they know a child is on a special diet, some will go to any length to tempt and tease him into eating something he shouldn't. Harris went through this hard experience. We found out how really cruel some children can be. They seem to sense the child is accomplishing something. They react with jealousy, temptation, and cruel words.

Take Henry for example: Every time he saw Harris in the school hall, sarcastically he would shout things like, "Hey, there's the kid who's on a crummy health diet! Yuck! He's still a dummy!"

Or take the case of Danny, who would flaunt his twinkies or ding dongs in Harris's face and say, "Umm... don't you wish you had some of this?"

Again, there were some children who actually tried to hide their goodies from Harris so he wouldn't be tempted. They were a true blessing to us.

If, at any time during this course of therapy, you want to know how your child is progressing, just ask his brother or sister. No one should know better.

Each time I asked Steven how Harris was progressing, he answered by demanding, "Keep him on his diet!" He saw more of an improvement in him than anyone. Steven was also a great source of encouragement.

Just as no single key opens all doors, no single person has all the answers to this problem. But keep searching and be open to other avenues. Relief sometimes comes in unexpected ways — often when things seem to be at their worse — so don't despair. The answers lie within the child's body. Interpreting the way his body expresses itself is a skill that must be learned and controlled if he is to enjoy what life has to offer. The fruits of that labor are good health and a sense of well-being.

# 6. Snack, Crackle, Flop

Nine-year-old Kevin strolled into the variety store, trying to be inconspicuous. He walked slowly to the candy section. There he began stashing candies into his pockets, eyeing the store carefully to make sure no one was watching. He left with several days' supply.

This was a typical event for Kevin. He had been stealing candy for several months, because of his addiction to sweets. Eventually, the inevitable happened. He was caught in the act. The police were called and his parents summoned.

Unknown to his parents, Kevin had been hiding his candy thefts behind the garage in a can he had buried. His mother could never understand why he wasn't hungry at mealtimes, or why he had such wide mood swings.

Many children like Kevin try to satisfy their "sweet tooth," only to find it can't be done. They are sugarholics. Their bodies merely crave more. Almost immediately after consuming sweets a child has a "sugar high," like alcohol to an alcoholic or drugs to an addict. The child feels good right away, but suffers the familiar drop within a few hours (nervousness, irritability, maniacal behavior, etc.).

A child's taste buds are not geared for extreme sweetness. Once refined sugar is removed from his diet, the child will notice that the craving starts to dwindle. His false "high" will be gone. His body will settle down. But once he eats another sugared goody, the trouble starts over. His restraint vanishes. His body begins to crave sugar once again. He feels he can't do without it.

Elimination of sugar alone from the diet can end some children's hyperactivity. No longer will there be uncontrolled, rapid absorption of sugar into the bloodstream. Parents then won't have to resort to drugs for control. Sugar elimination often can have the same desired effect as drug therapy, without the side effects.

## Remove Refined Sugars

It will be extremely difficult to place your child on a completely sugar-free diet, but if you want him to improve and break his emotional and physical ties to sugar, you will make the sacrifice. In fact, the whole family will benefit from this one change. They may complain and grumble about the disappearance of their sugared goodies, but your hyperactive child should show such a remarkable and welcome change that soon they will be thankful.

The positive effect of eliminating sugar from a hyperactive's diet is supported by much successful research and many pleased parents, as you will see in this book. This may not be the only solution to hyperactivity in some children, but it is a change that needs to be made. Even if you can't detect a change in the child (which is highly unlikely), do not let him have any sugar! There may be other conditions blocking improvement. Maximum benefits cannot be produced in one swift motion.

Refined sugar goes through a refining process that leaves it comprised of empty calories and nothing else. It offers no vitamins, minerals, or fiber. Consequently, sugar does absolutely nothing to help bodies grow strong and healthy. Because sugar does cause hyperactivity in many children, it should be the first item eliminated from the diet.

It is an unfortunate fact, however, that many children are pacified, bribed, rewarded, sympathized with, and apologized to with sugar. As a result, they have come to associate acceptance, love, and good behavior with sugar (the sugar-reward syndrome). Punishment often means denial of sugar. I recall vividly how I would promise Harris and Steven sweet treats if they would eat all their vegetables.

When sugar is eliminated from the child's diet, he should soon lose his craving. His behavior should improve, as my child's did. Meantime, you might prepare yourself for some strong objections from your child, but don't give in. When cravings pass, and he improves, you will breathe a sigh of grateful relief.

Take Joan as an example. She experienced hurt and humiliation when she removed the sugar from seven-year-old Danny's diet.

"Danny had refused to eat hardly anything but sugary foods. He was a raging monster." Joan said, "I replaced the sugar with wholesome foods, which at first he refused to eat. He often shouted, 'You're mean!' 'I hate you!' or 'I wish you weren't my mother!' He would run to his room and bang on the walls, screaming obscenities."

After eliminating sugar, Danny settled down. He made such an incredible transition, Joan added, "It was worth the agony!"

You're probably thinking that your child will sneak into the kitchen when you're not around and fill up on cookies, cake, candy, soft drinks, or other goodies. This may be true. Most hyperactive children, like Kevin, learn to be expert thieves. Therefore, you will be more successful if the whole family keeps no sweets for him to sneak. Then no one will be tempted. You will also soon discover luscious, sugar-free treats that everyone will enjoy.

Your friends and relatives may begin to wonder what new fad you're onto now. But once you begin solving the puzzle of your child's own body chemistry, they will know you are on the right track. Meanwhile, keep in mind that each small success makes life easier for everyone.

You will only be harming your child if you allow him to have an occasional sugar snack. I found that even one small infraction would cause a negative behavioral reaction from Harris for up to two days. Other parents have reported their problems lasting up to four days.

Ask yourself if it's worth it. Some parents think so — occasionally. Others strictly forbid it. They find that their child loses his ability to reason, and they can't cope with the erratic behavior.

### Pitter-Patter of Little Paws

Harris was eleven when we surprised him with a six-week-old puppy. He instantly labeled it Dino after the Flintstones' character. He showered it with love and attention.

Dino brought a ray of sunshine into our son's life. They became like Siamese twins. He took Dino everywhere. If Dino couldn't go, then he wouldn't go.

A week after Dino's arrival, we left on an Oregon vacation. Harris wanted Dino to go. He was full of promises to care for him so he wouldn't be any trouble.

Before leaving town, we stopped to stock up on ice. There on the store's counter, lay a candy bar. With his current charming personality and dancing blue eyes (and with Dino in hand), Harris pleaded convincingly for the candy bar. I bought it. He downed it in nothing flat.

An hour later, I regretted my moment of weakness. His temper flared. He wept, whined and wailed at the least provocation. We coaxed him to behave normally, but he grabbed Dino and held him close, as tears streamed down his cheeks.

"I keep kissing my puppy," he cried. "I love him so much. But he won't tell me he loves me too!"

This depression was the effect of one candy bar. Others were worse.

Pediatrician William G. Crook, M.D. says in his book *Can Your Child Read? Is He Hyperactive?*: "I've found that sugar is a major cause of hyperactivity in my own patients."[1]

Therefore, in all probability, you will discover, like us, that sugar does make a difference in the way your hyperactive child behaves.

If you are truly serious about wanting your child to get better, remove the sugar from his diet. It's a big step to take, but one that is necessary. I was extremely skeptical but found — it works!

Instead of a sweet treat, begin rewarding your child with money, a new toy, a special event or even a few minutes of your time.

For sweet snacks or desserts use only fruits. They should never be eaten without some form of good quality protein. The best and most common sources of protein foods are lean meat, fish, and poultry. Others are soy products, cheeses (only the natural ones should be eaten), wheat germ, nuts and seeds, and their butters, eggs, whole grains, legumes, and sprouts. These will ward off the up-and-down behavior, a familiar characteristic of the hyper child.

### List of Forbidden Sugars

| | |
|---|---|
| White Sugar: | Stripped of all nutrients; usually derived from sugar cane or sugar beet; full of calories, has no fiber. |
| Turbinado Sugar: | Sometimes called raw sugar; prepared from unrefined and unbleached crystals after the last molasses has been removed. |
| Brown Sugar: | White sugar with molasses added. |
| Yellow D Sugar: | Raw sugar with molasses added. |
| Corn Syrup: | Most corn syrup on the market is not pure, but has sugar (sucrose) syrup added. |
| Maple-Flavored Syrup: | A substitute for pure maple syrup, usually labeled as maple-flavored syrup. It usually contains corn syrup, water, refined sugar, artificial flavorings, colorings, and preservatives. |
| Fructose: | Called fruit sugar; a processed refined sugar. |

Any other refined sugar.

Rules to remember are: Never give a child sugar before bedtime. It will show in his behavior the next morning. Never give a child any form of sugar (refined or natural) on an empty stomach. If any form of sugar is eaten, it should be done so with a good source of quality protein.

Even Harris has learned to follow these rules, on his own. If, on a rare occasion, he does eat a forbidden sweet, he refuses to eat it on an empty stomach, even with persuasion from friends.

## List of Approved Substitutes

Many parents have found, as I have, that all forms of sweeteners have the same effect on their hyperactive child. The body can't distinguish among the sugars for energy. It merely converts them to glucose, or blood sugar. Even foods that are not normally thought of as being sweet contain a form of sugar. For instance: lactose, the sugar in milk; fructose, the sugar in fruits and honey; maltose, the sugar in corn.

If you still feel you occasionally must have some sweeteners in the house, fruit juice concentrates are a superior choice or one of the following sweeteners, but they should be kept to a bare minimum.

| | |
|---|---|
| Blackstrap Molasses: | Very strong-tasting; a by-product of sugar, the beet or cane syrup thrown off in the final spinning of the sugar refining process. Retains some beneficial elements, namely iron, calcium, and phosphorus, but also others. |
| Barbados Molasses: | Though made from sugar cane, it is a completely different product from blackstrap: a milder, dark-brown syrup, with lighter-tasting flavor than blackstrap. |
| Sorghum: | A syrup made from pure, sweet sorghum cane juice, similar in taste to light molasses or maple syrup. Only blackstrap molasses is richer in iron than sorghum. |
| Honey: | The most popular natural sweetener. Should be raw, unfiltered, unheated; Heating destroys nutrients. Comes in many flavors, depending on crop from which bees have collected their nectar. (It has been advised that children under age three not eat honey.) |
| Pure Maple Syrup: | Delicious and mild, but expensive. Derived from the sap of maple trees. |
| Barley Malt and Rice Syrup: | These are the cooked liquid of fermented grains. |

If you do use these sweeteners, do so sparingly. Gradually decrease the amount used. The child's taste for the sweetness will change. He will make the best headway if all sugars are totally eliminated.

Some children can tolerate a little occasionally, but not a large amount. Again, some parents find that if their child has only a mild reaction, it's worth the splurge — occasionally, not routinely.

From this choice of sweeteners, most choose honey. There are many different types, ranging from light and delicate to dark and strong. As a general rule, the darker the color, the stronger the taste. A few of the varieties to choose from are alfalfa, buckwheat (dark color, pungent flavor), clover (the most popular, with a mild flavor), orange-blossom, tupelo and others.

By experimenting, you can find one that's just right for your family's taste. Or, again, you might want to use different types for different purposes. When baking with honey, the oven temperature should be decreased 25 degrees, since honey tends to brown faster than other sweeteners.

In recipes that normally call for one cup of sugar, some suggest substituting ¾ cup of honey and then reduce liquid in the recipe by ¼ cup. But since honey has about twice the sweetening power as sugar, it's best to use only ½ cup honey.

I began reducing the amount called for in recipes and our tastes gradually began to change. Now I use less and hear no complaints.

Fruit or fruit juice concentrates as sweeteners really give home-baked items a delicious taste. Part fruit or fruit juice concentrate, and part honey would be good. Part molasses (although strong-tasting) gives home-baked items a different, yet delightful, flavor. With imaginative experimentation, the possibilities are endless. The important thing is not to overdo.

I have found that even some of the healthful candies made with nutritious, power-packed foods such as peanut butter, tahini, sesame or sunflower seeds, nuts, milk, wheat germ, etc., even though they contain high doses of nutrients, have entirely too much honey in them. It's best to avoid even them, in order to cut down on the amount of honey or any other sweetener your child is eating. If you have thrown out the refined sugars but are still eating nutritious foods with too much honey or sweetener, nothing is accomplished.

You may believe that your family doesn't eat much sugar, but it is included in many unsuspected foods. Until I began reading labels on every processed food, I didn't realize the downright sneaky places I would find it. Much to my surprise, it was in nearly every food we had been eating. Sugar is added to many foods as an inexpensive filler.

You will find sugar in boxed cereals and granolas (up to 31% sugar), canned soups, soft drinks, fruit-flavored drinks (usually 12% sugar), flavored gelatin (83% sugar), puddings, peanut butter, some canned vegetables such as corn (11% sugar), ketchup (29% sugar), mayonnaise, canned fruit, hot dogs, bologna, flavored yogurt, cakes, cookies, candies, jellies — and a long list of others, too numerous to name.

## Negative States

A multitude of obstacles will block the reshaping of your child's eating patterns. Though never planned, setbacks are part of our learning process. There will be many "sugar situations" with which your child will need to cope: TV's influence — daily brainwashing by sugar commercials; probably the hardest to escape, peer pressure, relatives — raised eyebrows, open criticism directed at you for "depriving" your child, movies, shopping, parties, holidays, to name a few.

Traditionally, holidays bring an explosion of sugar-laden goodies. They are literally shoved upon the child. These obstacles have to be dealt with by discovering clever, satisfying ways to resolve them.

Halloween, which revolves around candy, is one of our obstacles. It is a time of joy for many, with jack-o-lanterns in the windows, hanging dime store decorations all around, visits to haunted houses, parties, sharing spooky ghost stories, and treats that lure the tricksters. But, for those who have to forego the treats, it can be full of temptation, heartbreak, envy, and tears.

This is what we do: I let Harris go trick-or-treating and collect the candy. Then we buy it from him at so much for each piece, sometimes its true worth, sometimes more. He then is able to purchase a long-awaited toy or other desired prize.

Of course, the best thing to do is to have the child forego trick-or-treating altogether, but I could never deny Harris the fantasy of dressing up in his imaginative costume and the adventure of going from door to door with his comrades.

If your child does go out, be sure and feed him well beforehand. Then the temptation to eat candy will not be so overwhelming. Some parents let their children choose only one or two pieces of candy. Whichever method you choose, get the candy out of the child's sight as quickly as possible.

Another obstacle is birthday parties. They are a difficult time for Harris. They usually cause much fussing, fighting, chaos, and tears. Harris is unable to handle the over-excitement. Some parents of hyperactive children find it best to forego parties. I belong to this group.

If Harris is invited to a party, we usually just send a gift. We then make it up to him by purchasing him a small gift. When his birthday rolls around, I estimate how much we would have spent on party decorations, prizes, goodies, etc., and give him that amount of money. Then he is able to purchase something he wants or just keep it for pocket money. This works well with Harris.

There may be certain occasions such as birthdays or holidays, when you feel it is worth your suffering to let your child eat something he shouldn't. You may have to live with the reminder of his wrongful eating for several days. A lot may depend on the severity of his problems, as well as what you may be willing to endure.

However, if he does eat a forbidden food, it should be eaten on Friday evening or Saturday, so the effects wear off before school on Monday.

## Hypoglycemia

The term hypoglycemia, simply translated, means low blood sugar. When a child eats a meal high in sugars or starches (which convert to sugar), it leads to an excess of glucose in the blood within a few hours. The pancreas over-responds to the sugar, and produces too much insulin. The body then overreacts, trying to get rid of the excess glucose, and the blood sugar drops below normal fasting level.

Glucose is needed by the brain for proper functioning. When the blood doesn't supply an adequate amount, symptoms occur, signaling the body to raise the blood sugar level. They are: incessant hunger, nervousness, irritability, exhaustion, dizziness, tremor, weakness, depression, drowsiness, headaches, mental confusion, antisocial behavior, inability to concentrate, muscle aches, prolonged sleepiness, incoherent speech, maniacal behavior, crying spells, forgetfulness, unprovoked anxieties, phobias, and others.

Many hyperactive children are hypoglycemic. Ordinary sweets are a real hazard to their brain and nervous system. This often complicates the job of tracking down other factors responsible for their condition. For one who craves sugar, a five hour glucose tolerance test (some doctors suggest a six hour test) will confirm hypoglycemia. An alert doctor can detect the symptoms without having to administer a glucose tolerance test. Changes in the blood sugar affect behavior!

Hypoglycemia is a highly controversial medical condition. Some doctors agree it is very common, though one that often is misdiagnosed and mistreated. Still other doctors — perhaps a majority — disagree. They do acknowledge the condition exists, but contend it is not common.

As the body attempts to get the glucose level back up to normal, the child experiences a voracious craving for sweets. But eating more sugar only triggers the cycle all over again. Sugar aggravates, rather than improves, the hypoglycemic condition. Contrary to what one might think, the solution to low blood sugar is not eating more sugar. The only way to correct the condition is to take him off the "drug" sugar.[3] The idea is to control the production of insulin and keep the blood sugar on an even keel.

If your child is hypoglycemic, the first step is to follow a low-carbohydrate, high-protein diet. He should eat smaller, more frequent meals consisting of high-quality protein.

The protein foods do not trigger the overabundant insulin-release. They release sugar into the bloodstream slowly. The blood sugar then does not drop so dramatically low after eating. If he nibbles on protein foods, the craving for sugar will pass.

Here is an example — the success story of eight-year-old Ronnie. His mother said, "He was an awful mischief-maker. He existed in a yo-yo manner. At times he was cheerful, then he would turn into a wretched little beast, red-faced with fury, yelling at the top of his lungs."

The doctor said Ronnie had low blood sugar and advised them to remove the sugar from his diet. He was to eat plenty of high-protein foods and more vegetables.

"Almost instantly, we began to see results," Kay said. "Ronnie's disposition improved, as well as his school grades. He was like a new child. His sugar cravings soon disappeared."

When asked what he felt was the most important improvement due to his diet change, Ronnie excitedly answered, "This is the first time I've had a lot of friends."

"That's why," Kay said, "he is willing to remain on his sugar-free diet."

Sugar elimination is the first important step on the road to success. It's a tough step, but the first step is usually the hardest. Success is bound to follow.

# 7. Forward Movement

The year Harris began kindergarten proved disastrous, as predicted. We had not yet tackled his hyperactivity through a changed diet. With Harris's boundless energy, his schoolteacher found he was unable to sit still, take directions, concentrate, or do his schoolwork.

Harris was blessed with a kind, gentle, understanding teacher. She had the patience of a saint with a high frustration level for her little people. Just to watch the way she lovingly handled each one was heartwarming. As she told fairy tales each day, her eyes grew huge and her hands waved as she dramatized each verse.

Harris instantly fell in love with her.

About halfway through the school year, Harris still had not mastered his ABC's like the rest of the group. It was obvious that the only way he would pass was for me to teach him. I spent two hours daily on the task. He was slow, his attention span zero, and he became frustrated quickly. My frustrations grew along with his.

I didn't realize then that the wisest thing I could have done would have been to let him stay back an extra school year. But I wanted him to remain with the new acquaintances he had made this first tough school year.

Dr. Agatha M. Thrash of Alabama says that placing a child in a grade level he barely qualifies for in terms of age frequently leads to trouble, and that hyperactive children are usually immature in their personality and mental development. She recommends they start school late. Little boys are much more vulnerable than girls, she says, because they mature less rapidly.

This was the same year the Feingold Diet book surfaced, making national headlines, declaring that diet made a difference in the lives of hyperactive children. Harris's teacher borrowed the book from the library and thrust it at me when I came in one morning to help in the classroom. She remarked that she felt I needed it.

I took the new book home and leafed through it, not feeling too enthusiastic. I thought the diet would be time-consuming, confusing, restrictive and above all, frustrating. Silently I talked myself out of it by saying that I had a hyperactive, learning-disabled child on my hands. I had no time for a special diet! Besides, why try something I was sure would fail?

The next day I returned the book with a "Thank you, but no thanks!" which meant, "I have better ways to spend my time!"

It wasn't until five years later, that I realized I should have heeded the clever teacher's suggestion. During those years, tutors were hired, cutting into our already-low budget. Harris spent hours after school catching up on work. Time from my own busy schedule was spent at home trying to help him keep up with the rest of his peer group. There was little success. All the while, he was barely passing with C's and D's. He continued to grow worse mentally, physically, and academically.

## Feingold — Here We Come!

The late Ben Feingold, M.D., an allergist and pediatrician at Kaiser-Permanente Medical Center, San Francisco, was the first to connect food additives and hyperactive behavior. He developed his diet theory in 1973 — commonly referred to as "The Feingold Diet." It consisted of removing artificial flavors, colors, and preservatives from a hyperactive child's diet and, for some children, the substances called salicylates, which occur naturally in some foods. He wrote a book (*Why Your Child Is Hyperactive,* Random House, 1974) in which he expounded on his experiences.

Dr. Feingold found that at least half the hyperactive children who go on the rigid diet and stick to it show a dramatic change in behavior. They become more relaxed, happy, and contented. Their school performance also improves dramatically. But he found that if a child eats only two forbidden foods twice a week, it might totally eliminate any good results for that week.

Dr. Feingold was bombarded from all sides. Some worked toward disproving his theory, others worked toward confirming it. Still, his theory has neither been proved nor disproved by the FDA.

It did, however, launch a fresh approach in dealing with hyperkinesis, and was unquestionably a tremendous step in the right direction. There are many parents nationwide who have touted the successful results from the diet. In fact, the Feingold Association is comprised mainly of families who use and uphold the diet.

## Piecing Together the Puzzle

The life of a hyperactive child is complex, like a giant complicated puzzle with many pieces. To solve it, one must find all the pieces and use them correctly.

The child's life, itself, is a puzzle. At times it seems the puzzle will never fit together. The elimination of sugar is one piece to this puzzle. The Feingold Diet is another one.

Let's say that the outside edge of the puzzle is the child's body chemistry. It might seem best for the border to be put together first, so the platform can be set to interpret the limits. In like fashion, the child's body chemistry determines the limits. If certain ingredients are not in their proper places, in the right amount, at the right time, the body will fail to function properly.

In the early stages, the puzzle seems to be a real mess. None of the pieces seem to fit. But one gradually begins placing the pieces together where they should be. And some seem to automatically fall into place as one goes along.

*You, as a parent, are the only one who can accept the responsibility of solving your child's own puzzle. You can put the pieces all together and make it work.* You are the only one who loves and cares for him enough to take the time. And you are the only one who is with him enough to gain by doing so.

## Nutrient Connection

It is vitally important to supply a child's body with the nutrients it needs. Sound nutrition is essential to produce vibrant health. The brain, the organ that controls a child's behavior and ability to learn, needs a constant, steady source of glucose for fuel. Any substantial increase or decrease in the amount of available glucose can result in malfunctioning of the brain.

Sound nutrition directly influences a child's ability to think, learn, and retain information, his mood and temperament, his mental alertness and stability. Nutrition affects social development and other behavioral patterns, resistance to disease, allergies, and the speed of wound healing. Good nutrition is needed for good digestion and assimilation, physical development (bone structure, teeth and dental caries, hair, nails, complexion, strength) and many other functions as well.

Optimal good health is related to diet as much as to environment or heredity. A child in poor health is more vulnerable to diseases. They will invade the body like weeds in an unkept garden.

I didn't know what impact food had on health, but I was learning fast.

## Puzzle Pieces: Exclusion of Milk

I ran into my friend, Brenda, in our health food store in 1979. Her child, seven-year-old Melinda, had been on the Feingold Diet for quite some time.

She mentioned that she had read Dr. Lendon Smith's book *Improving Your Child's Behavior Chemistry,* in which he claims that sugar can interfere with normal blood sugar levels and cause behavioral problems. He also blames milk for physical and behavioral problems in many individuals.

Brenda had withdrawn sugar from Melinda's diet. She then withdrew the milk.

"The results were phenomenal!" she said.

The thought of excluding milk and milk products from a child's diet shocked me. I couldn't imagine any child not having milk — especially Harris. After all, it was considered to be such a good food. I couldn't see how milk could have anything to do with hyperactive behavior.

I was strongly opposed to taking Harris off milk and milk products. Besides, I reasoned, they were his favorite foods!

But we reached a standstill where he simply was not making headway. I hesitantly took the final step — I eliminated milk products. He made an astounding improvement, as if he had been sedated. Even his teacher noticed a big change in his behavior and schoolwork — almost overnight. This once-flustered parent was very relieved.

Harris's grades had been nothing to brag about. All his tests were usually right around the seventy mark. Shortly after I excluded milk from his diet, he began studying diligently for his "States and Capitals" test in fifth grade. The test was hard. He had to match all the capitals with the states on one sheet of paper and match the states with the capitals on the next. Then he had to write each state and capital on the map.

For several hours each day all week, he sprawled on the floor with his books strewn all around.

The day the test results came in, he bounded in the door.

"Mom," he said calmly, trying to contain himself. "I failed my test."

My heart almost stopped beating. For once I was at a loss for comforting, reassuring words . . .

Then his eyes lit up and he exuberantly announced the truth, "I made a hundred!"

He was one of three children who had made a hundred!

After Harris had been off milk for awhile, I decided to introduce it back into his diet. I wanted to be doubly sure. He experienced an awful reaction. He lay on the floor kicking and screaming, having a fit. He also began to harass Steven verbally. His fits and harassment persisted off and on for two days. Those were two long and miserable days for all of us.

As time passed, I continued to reintroduce milk into his diet several more times to be positively sure. After all, I didn't want to judge his sensitivity to anything as important as milk by merely a few trials.

I appeared to be quite stubborn. Once again I asked myself, "Why me?" Why does my child have to be sensitive to milk? So commonly consumed and added to so many other foods, it's considered to be the near-perfect food. Why is Harris sensitive to a food he enjoys so much, and that supplies the calcium and other nutrients his body needs?

Milk is a very common cause of adverse reactions in hyperactive children. Some adverse reactions are allergic in nature, but some may result from a non-allergic intolerance to milk, or the milk sugar, lactose.

It is often difficult to distinguish between food intolerances and food allergies. Many intolerances are considered to be an allergy, when actually they are not. Linda Clark distinguishes between allergies and intolerances in *The Handbook of Natural Remedies for Common Ailments*.[1] An allergen may exist in the food and an intolerance may lie in the person.

Milk intolerance is very common. The symptoms are stomach cramps, bloating, gas, diarrhea, nausea or vomiting, mucous, nasal symptoms, headaches, heartburn, fatigue, and constipation.

Millions of people cannot tolerate lactose, the milk sugar present in cow's milk, or products made from it.[2] Babies apparently are born with an enzyme, called lactase, which helps the body to accept lactose in milk. But, after weaning, the lactase enzyme seems to disappear for the rest of their lives.

People who tolerate milk past infancy are the abnormal ones, and not the other way around. The word is out that we are actually healthier if we don't consume milk products (there are many other good sources of calcium). Many doctors believe that milk is a detrimental food.[3]

Some experts recommend its total exclusion. Others recommend no more than two glasses daily.

One of Harris's doctors suggested that perhaps his body could handle only a small amount of milk at a time — such as two ounces. In fact, many doctors do advise that if a person has a milk intolerance, he does not have to steer completely clear of milk. Although milk-intolerant people cannot handle large amounts well, they can sometimes manage with smaller amounts.

Furthermore, they experience less trouble if they ingest milk with meals rather than by itself. It is also advised not to drink cold milk — which seems to cause more trouble than warm milk — on an empty stomach.

Milk and dairy products are promoted primarily for their calcium content — for strong bones and teeth. But surprisingly enough, it has been discovered that those who drink milk and are intolerant to it, seem to have trouble assimilating the milk's calcium. Consequently, they may develop a calcium deficiency.

To test your child's tolerance, milk and all milk products (including goat's milk) should be left out of the child's diet for three to four weeks. They may then be added back to see what kind of a reaction occurs. *Cow's milk is one of the most common causes of hyperactivity in children.* The question, "What foods are most commonly involved in causing hyperactivity and other nervous system allergies?" is answered by Dr. Crook in *Can Your Child Read? Is He Hyperactive?*

"Cow's milk and chocolate (including cola) perhaps lead the list of foods which produce allergic symptoms in school-age children,"[4] says Dr. Crook.

If you need to eliminate cow's milk from your child's diet, soybean milk is the usual substitute. But some children may be sensitive to that also.

Dianne, the mother of an eight-year-old son, says, "When I give Bud milk, he is cranky, aggressive, and wets the bed. It's as obvious as if he wore a sign advertising that he drank milk."

Helen says her ten-year-old son, Sam, refuses outright to drink milk on the grounds that it makes him act "wild and crazy."

If your child does have an adverse reaction to milk and it has to be excluded from his diet, he must take calcium supplements, along with other necessary vitamin and mineral supplements. (For guidance, refer to the Mineral section in Appendix C.)

Some milk-sensitive children eat beef without reaction. However, since cow's milk and beef come from the same animal (as with eggs and chicken), it might be wise to exclude beef from his diet for a week or so. You can then add it back to see what kind of a reaction occurs.

Alexander Schauss conducted a controlled study, relating diet to delinquency. The detailed study is in his published book, *Diet, Crime and Delinquency,* which is enlightening. The study reveals that chronic juvenile offenders drink twice as much milk as non-offenders.[5] Thus experts believe that milk might actually play a role in delinquency. When the amount of milk is cut down, the children's behavioral problems are reduced.

This is not to say that milk is not a highly nutritious food, but rather that many individuals cannot tolerate it or have an allergy to it.

Sensitivity to a particular food should not normally be diagnosed on the basis of only one trial. The child could have a mild cold or upset stomach which coincided with the new food. Therefore, if there is no reaction when you reintroduce milk, you may then add the natural white cheeses (Swiss, monterey jack, or mozzarella). You can find uncolored cheddar cheese at health food stores. These cheeses, if they are safe for your child to eat, are always good as a snack, and are an excellent source of protein, calcium, magnesium, and other nutrients.

## Chocolate Disaster

Chocolate is another common problem food. It causes adverse reactions in many hyperactive children. Chocolate is a particularly bad allergy food and may to some degree affect as many as twelve million Americans.[6]

Chocolate can make a child tired, angry, irritable and upset, leading to temper tantrums, destructive behavior, depression, and violence.

Chocolate usually is combined with sugar (40%). Together, they can be so disastrous to a hyperactive child's system that chocolate should be entirely eliminated from the child's diet. Likewise with the cola products, like cola soft drinks. Chocolate and cola are members of the same food family, deriving from the cola nut.

Furthermore, there are nutritional drawbacks to chocolate. It contains caffeine and interferes with calcium absorption. The worst problem, perhaps, is the large number of people who are allergic to chocolate. It is second on the list of allergenic foods. The allergy frequently is a subtle one that goes unrecognized. Paradoxically, the allergy can take the form of a craving.

## Carob: A Natural Treat

There is a delicious alternative to chocolate, called carob, a much better choice and a natural treat for everyone. The taste and appearance is remarkably similar, although carob has a milder, more subtle flavor. Carob is not bitter like chocolate, so there is no need to add sugar or milk. It is already rich in natural sugar.

Carob contains many trace minerals, as well as fibers and pectin. Unlike chocolate, it has no caffeine. Carob is often called St. John's bread, because some scholars believe that carob sustained John the Baptist in the wilderness. However, since carob is a member of the legume family, which includes peas and beans, a child who is sensitive to legumes may also be sensitive to carob.

## Wipe Out Whites

Dr. Smith found that refined white flour in a child's diet can interfere with normal blood sugar levels, causing behavioral problems. White flour has been refined, which actually means "robbed" of natural fiber and nutrients. Therefore, white flour products and refined white rice should be eliminated.

In the refining process, the outer coating of a wheat kernel or the bran is removed. Since the bran is the highest fiber-containing portion of the wheat, white flour can make a child's elimination sluggish. The wheat germ, which contains protein, vitamins and minerals (especially the B's and E) is also removed during refining. The coarser parts of the endosperm, also high in fiber and protein, are eliminated. The end product is a clear flour of a creamy color. This goes through a bleaching process, all of which leaves the white flour depleted of precious nutrients. Then synthetic vitamins are added so it can be called "enriched."

Always look for the one-hundred percent stone-ground whole wheat flour. The whole grain flours contain all fiber, vitamins and minerals removed in the refining process. Whole wheat flour has more protein, more vitamins and minerals, and less carbohydrate than white flour. Stone-ground indicates that it has been exposed to the least possible heat in the grinding process, which maintains its high nutritional content.

It is best to keep whole grains refrigerated or frozen for longer periods of storage, so they won't get rancid or spoiled. I keep mine in the freezer, taking out what I need for the week. I purchase whole grains in bulk quantities. Our refrigerator won't hold them all.

Higher oil content makes whole grains more perishable than refined grains. If you are unable to keep your whole grains refrigerated or in the freezer, then opt for a cool dry place in tightly sealed containers.

If your family is used to eating white flour, you may have to gradually include whole grain flours until they adapt. Some start out by using half whole-grain flour and half unbleached white flour. Families seem to adjust better this way. But the complete change to whole grains should be made immediately for your child's earlier improvement.

Some children may be sensitive or allergic to all grains — wheat, corn, rye, oats, barley or rice, all "kin" to each other. The same goes for the citrus family — lemon, lime, grapefruit, orange, tangerine, tangelo, citric acid — and the legume family — peas, peanuts, beans, soybeans, etc.

Sometimes, if one grain isn't tolerated well, others can be. But if your child is sensitive to one or more grains, you will want to use the other grains sparingly so he won't become sensitive to them.

## Bushel of Trouble

If your child is sensitive to citrus fruits, they should be avoided. However, if one citrus fruit isn't tolerated well, another one might be. If your child is sensitive to all citrus fruits, you will want to compensate with Vitamin C supplements or other sources. Vitamin C is required daily and is easily obtained in citrus fruits.

In general, it's best for a child to eat the whole fruit rather than drink the fruit juice. It takes longer, provides fiber, and is more satisfying to the body. While fruit juice is undeniably delicious, it is far better to let a child quench his thirst with a piece of fruit. Nature provides a balance of nutrients in the whole fruit that is lacking in the juice.

## Eggs

Eggs can cause an adverse reaction in hyperactive children, but it is usually a true allergic reaction. Eggs do not have to be avoided at this time unless you are suspicious that your child might be allergic to them.

## Junk Food Trap

Junk food simply means empty calories . . . foods full of fat, sugar, salt, food flavors, colors, and other additives. They are relatively low in nutrients for the large number of calories they contain.

Junk food and sugar raise the blood sugar. The body then puts out insulin to drive the blood sugar down. This causes the adrenal gland to attempt to stabilize the blood sugar by pouring out adrenal hormones. This causes rapid heartbeat, an increase in blood pressure, breathing problems, and muscle tension.

Generally, some of the items classified as junk foods are: coffee, tea and alcohol; refined sugared goodies — ice cream, candy, cakes, pies, cookies and doughnuts; soft drinks, especially cola drinks and powdered drinks; foods that are refined, processed, highly salted, fried and fatty; potato chips and other salty snacks; packaged dry cereals; so-called "convenience" packaged foods; foods at fast-food places — you get the picture.

Dr. Thrash states that many of the hyperactive children who have been studied have finicky eating habits. They are unwilling to eat fruits and vegetables, and want mainly milk, cheese, boxed cereals, crackers, and white bread — just what they shouldn't be eating.

Harris should be in the Guinness Book of World Records for being the pickiest eater of all times! He doesn't want anything green to ever pass his lips, except — of all things — avocado.

It's not easy to persuade a child to eat a piece of fruit or a healthy snack when he really wants a doughnut or a piece of candy. It's also difficult to fight the influence of alluring TV commercials and peer pressure.

Therefore, the earlier a child starts on wholesome foods, the better. It is difficult to break a life-long habit of twinkies, ding dongs, and soft drinks. When a child starts early he will grow up demanding wholesome foods, and be less likely to have faulty nutrition.

A good point is made by Dr. Smith in his book *Feed Your Kids Right*: "If school authorities want to stop discipline problems and vandalism in the classroom, they must do away with sugar and junk foods in the halls and close the candy stores within two miles of the school."[7]

## Other Substances

Substances other than food and food additives can also cause behavioral and/or physical problems in the hyperactive child. Therefore, it's a good idea to keep a close watch on the chemical odors, vapors and fumes in his environment. These could include tobacco smoke, synthetic fabrics, cooking and heating gas, substances around new construction (including insulation), cleaning agents, perfumes, animal dander, house dust or molds, gasoline fumes, auto exhaust, etc.

Fourteen-year-old Mark is an example. He flew into a frenzy while helping his parents paint their bedroom. He began acting like one of the Three Stooges, then his agitated activity increased. He began screaming and trying to fight with his younger sister and parents. The doctor said Mark was allergic to the paint. Mark's parents, however, were skeptical. A month later, upon painting another bedroom, a similar episode took place, and they knew.

## Each Child is Unique

How simple it would be if all hyperactive children were exactly the same! There would be no surprises and we would know well in advance just what to expect. Unfortunately, no two hyperactive children are the same. Each has his own unique biochemistry, so what works well with one child will not necessarily work the same with another.

Some specialists claim that the kind of brain chemistry that reacts to food additives may be present in only some hyperactive children. This could be true. No one knows for sure. I know that Harris reacts to food additives in his diet. I also know that many other parents find their hyperactive children also react to additives. (For list of additives, refer to Appendix A.)

This leads me to believe that additives do affect hyperactive children — possibly some children more than others. Who really knows? Even the experts disagree. One research finds they do. Another research disputes this claim. I do know, however, that leaving additives out of Harris's diet can't hurt him.

*The Natural Way Program* is different from the conventional treatment with drugs. Consequently, it must be fully carried out if parents do not want to resort to drugs.

## In Essence

*The Natural Way Program* consists of two phases:

1. An all natural food diet
   a. Foods to avoid
   b. Foods to eat
2. Vitamin and Mineral Therapy

Even though the program is an all-natural food diet, there are still some natural foods that should be eliminated at the beginning. They may be tried at a later date.

You may notice (as I did) that your child has an adverse reaction to two entirely different foods, but that one reaction is worse than the other. For instance, Harris had a more unfavorable reaction to sugar and milk than to some food additives. Some food additives — such as red dye — produced a worse reaction than others.

With some successful results the child should improve, if not become completely symptom-free. Life will then be easier for everyone. His family will be able to *like* him as well as *love* him. Best of all, he will feel he *can win*! This makes any child's life happier, more enjoyable and more complete!

To accomplish these goals, you will have to begin reading food labels.

# 8. Newsworthy Label

By now you may be shaking your head in total confusion. "How on earth do I understand what I read on labels?" you may ask.

My friend Rita experienced similar puzzlement when she began to improve her son Chad's learning problems through diet. She was stumped.

"What do I look for on a label? How can I tell the good guys from the bad guys?"

When I joined the rank of *label readers* I was confused, too. I was in store for a great number of surprises, but this was the beginning of success.

You'll find label readers in all the food store aisles. In fact, one of them might be Harris. He trails up and down the aisles, reading the labels on every food that looks good. This way, he can make certain he isn't missing out on any of the "good" foods he is allowed to eat. Interestingly enough, he sometimes discovers things I miss. When he does, his eyes twinkle and a big grin crosses his face at having outsmarted Mom.

## Natural Hoax

Keep in mind that, just because a food product has the word "natural" on it, it may not be an "all-natural" product. The word "natural" actually means, "in a state provided by nature, without man-made changes, not artificial or manufactured." But using the word "natural" is sometimes the food industry's way of evading consumer distrust of factory-made foods, so "natural" has come to mean whatever the manufacturer chooses for it to mean. That can be very different from what the consumer thinks it means. In plain words, food manufacturers may try to fool us by flaunting the word "natural," which is often far from being the truth. Careful reading pays.

Read all the label. Not part of it. If it takes a while to read, then move on to another product. Anything that's natural shouldn't take that long to discover. If a product really is natural, you will know it before wasting your time reading through words you don't understand.

Remember, the manufacturers are out for the almighty dollar, but you are after optimal health. It is not always an easy route, but a very rewarding one. We need to build health and prevent disease. By preventing disease, we can avoid struggling with cure or control, or medical treatment of symptoms.

Due to greater public awareness, a slight reduction has resulted in the use of chemical food additives. This goes to prove that there is power in what the public wants. Yet, sugar still is omnipresent. When we purchase these health-destroying products, we are, in effect, telling the manufacturers their products are acceptable. In other words, if he sells it, it has to be good. Right?

The consumer, in fact, is being conned. Some manufacturers seem to consider "What you don't know won't hurt you" their slogan. It does take knowledge to be consumers without being consumed. A new beginning, through a natural food diet, depends upon a willingness to learn.

Manufacturers contribute heavily to research in nutrition, trying to persuade the public that their products are harmless. As long as there are misconceptions about what is involved in a proper diet, their health-destroying foods will continue to do a booming business. We are paying the real price — healthwise. But, if their denatured, sugar- and chemical-laden foods don't sell, they no longer will be produced. Pass the word.

## Understand Labels

It is somewhat difficult to read labels at first. Some can be tricky. But, like eating, sleeping, or breathing, it soon becomes an unconscious habit. Foods are not always what they appear to be, so we must learn to read and understand the label.

Sugar is often listed as the number one ingredient on food labels. This means that that particular food has more sugar in it than any other ingredient. In other words, you are paying mostly for sugar.

Ingredients are labeled, generally, in descending order of volume in the product. Manufacturers, however, try to fool us in regard to the amount of sugar contained in their product. They will divide the sweetener into categories, to avoid listing it as the main ingredient. For example: the ingredients may be listed as "flour, brown sugar, honey, etc." It appears that flour is the major ingredient, but the combination of brown sugar and honey make sweeteners the overwhelming ingredient. Some manufacturers may even have three or four different sweetening agents.

It is important to read the label for additives and sugar on every tiny thing, regardless of how insignificant it might seem, such as toothpaste, mouthwash, vitamin supplements, canned goods, etc.

I thought toothpaste would be safe, until I read the labels on various brands. Ingredients may include artificial sweeteners, such as saccharin or sorbitol; preservatives; artificial flavors and colors. Some of the ingredients are really tongue twisters. The health food stores have a variety of natural ones.

One rule to follow: If you are in doubt about using a particular product — *don't*. I found it better to be safe than sorry.

Harris used to have an average of three bouts or more of bronchitis each winter and double that number of colds. He coughed constantly. To alleviate some of the soreness in his throat, he sucked on cough drops throughout the day.

When I went for a conference with his third grade schoolteacher, she remarked that she thought the cough drops were making him hyperactive. Again, out of ignorance, I paid little attention to her comment. Years later, when I became a label reader, I realized she was right. Cough drops are nothing more than candy.

Read the label on everything — even cough drops.

When purchasing flavor extracts buy only the "pure" extracts, such as "pure vanilla" or "pure lemon." They must have the word "pure" on the label. This means the flavor comes from that particular fruit or nut, instead of synthetic additives.

## What's in a Name?

When Harris first started on *The Natural Way Program,* I searched the health food stores for some wieners and bologna without the usual additives. I found that this type of products sold in health food stores experienced labeling problems with the U.S.D.A. It seems the Department of Agriculture will not let them call their products "hot dog," "frank" or "weiner" unless they add nitrites or nitrates to these meats. One particular food company said since they refuse to use these questionable chemicals, they are forced to use strange names such as, for wieners, "uncured cooked sausage... with wiener flavoring added." The food company said they actually don't use any flavoring, or any other additives. Their products contain only one-hundred percent meat and natural spices.

Since words like these can often be misleading — even though in a favorable way — it's always best to read the entire label, no matter where you purchase the product. Read the full list of ingredients, not just the front label.

But I do want to caution you. Since you will be preferring meats and other food products that don't have any preservatives, it won't be safe to keep them more than a few days in the refrigerator. They must be kept frozen and taken out as you need them.

The Food and Drug Administration says ketchup cannot be called ketchup unless it contains refined sugar. Consequently, some food companies have to call their honey-sweetened ketchup "Imitation" ketchup. If your child must eat ketchup, try to make your own or get honey-sweetened ketchup.

When a label has words we don't understand, we shouldn't purchase the product. A good rule to keep in mind is: "If God made it and man didn't change it, you can eat it. If you can't pronounce it, don't buy it."

# 9. Diet Diary

Are you confused? Overwhelmed? Are you wondering how you will ever manage to keep all this straight besides trying to figure out what works for your child and what doesn't?

Answer: Begin keeping records.

Thirty minutes after Harris drank a small glass of grape juice, he flew into a rage. He tried to demolish his room, breaking, smashing and tearing anything he could grab. At the time, I didn't realize he had a sensitivity to grapes. I specifically identified this culprit. It was easy. Others were not. Some I had to search for a month or more before the culprit was identified.

I could have simplified matters if I had taken the advice of my friend, Joyce. She kept records on her child. She told me to record every food Harris ate each day at the time he ate it, for several weeks or more until I could pinpoint the troublemakers.

It's hard to keep straight all the foods the child eats, besides trying to figure out what works and what doesn't. Therefore, the best solution is to take Joyce's advice. Keep records of his progress, best done by keeping a "diet diary."

I know what you're thinking. This will seem like a great deal of trouble, but you have nothing to lose except a little time. You have much to gain, however, in discovering the various foods that "set off" your child. This is how I finally pinpointed all the foods Harris could not eat. If they had all been as obvious as the grape juice, it would have been easy. His progress would have been faster if I had heeded Joyce's advice in the first place.

Of course, it seems easier to pop a pill (like Ritalin or Cylert) into the child and forget the diet altogether. But if a child has food allergies, food sensitivities, hypoglycemia, nutritional deficiencies, or other biochemical problems, they will continue or grow worse if his diet remains the same, even though the drugs help temporarily.

For example: Jeff's mother was killed in a car accident when he was nine years old. This left his dad, Ray, to raise the boy alone. Jeff became spoiled. His father let him have his own way to compensate for having lost his mother.

In earlier years, Jeff was labeled as hyperactive with learning problems. He began to grow worse. He became wild, mean and aggressive, with frequent outbursts of temper, wide mood swings. He often got into fist fights and did poorly in school. His attention span was zero. He also was clumsy and unable to do fine work with his hands.

Jeff had a lot of sugar, cola drinks, dry sugar-coated cereals, other junky foods — and milk. Cola drinks and doughnuts were common breakfast fare.

Close friends and relatives convinced Ray that Jeff needed help. Dr. Pierce, a neighbor, wrote a Cylert prescription for Jeff. He calmed down dramatically and began improving in school. Other problems began to surface, however. Jeff was often ill with colds, ear infections, headaches, vomiting and other stomach upsets. He complained of leg cramps. He had nightmares, wet the bed frequently, and was constantly thirsty.

Ray's boss became upset because Ray took off work so much to care for his sick child. The boss pressed Ray to take Jeff to a good pediatrician to reach the root of his problems.

Dr. Grant was tops in the pediatric field. He took blood tests and performed extensive examinations. He found that Jeff was anemic, hypoglycemic, and under-nourished. An allergist then found that Jeff could not tolerate sugar, milk, wheat, corn, peanuts, potatoes and red dye.

Ray was told, in essence, to clear their pantry of all food additives, sugar and junk food and to throw them in the garbage can. He did so. Jeff experienced withdrawal symptoms of irritability, restlessness, and violent behavior for three days. On the fourth day, to Ray's amazement, Jeff's behavior improved markedly.

Ray also began giving him supplemental vitamins and minerals. After awhile, Jeff's leg cramps disappeared. He no longer wet the bed. Colds and ear infections and stomach distresses disappeared. Jeff was calm and healthy.

Without this action, Jeff might still be on Cylert, with the drug only masking his symptoms.

## Keep Notes

It's important to write down every bite of food, beverage — whatever your child eats each day. Write beside it his behavior, whether good or bad, after eating each particular food. Even the small bites of food you might think don't count should be written down.

Is the child unruly, overactive, irritable, talking too much or having crying spells? Or is he calm, amiable, easy to get along with? It's easy for me to tell with Harris. He flies into a rage when he eats the wrong thing, like grape juice.

You will notice that certain foods do seem to set your child off. Or you may notice a decrease in the number of times he misbehaves. By this diet diary, you will be able to tell exactly which food is the culprit. You will have the solid evidence you need in black and white to determine what works and what doesn't.

At first I found myself reluctant to keep a diet diary. I didn't think I could accomplish anything, even though Joyce assured me it worked. But it proved to be more than worth the trouble.

A hyperactive child usually eats vast amounts of food and stays thin as a rail. Consequently, one's memory doesn't work too well, when it comes to remembering what he ate from one meal to the next, or from one snack to the next. Harris seems to eat one continuous meal all day long, like trying to fill a bottomless stomach. It was impossible to remember everything without keeping the diary.

## Recruiting Help

It will be crucial to inform your child's schoolteacher of what you're doing. You will need his or her help. You might explain what you're doing and why. Let the teacher know what progress you hope to accomplish from it — such as having a calmer and more manageable child. Ask the teacher to keep an eye on what the child eats at school. He should be taking his super-nutritious foods to school, but children often swap lunches.

The teacher will be concerned about your child's progress and will probably be more than willing to help. Life will be easier for the teacher if just one hyperactive child settles down. There can be five or six hyperactive children in one classroom. The year Harris started his diet, he was in fifth grade. There were five hyperactive children in the classroom — all boys.

When I first began keeping Harris's diet diary, his teacher began keeping notes at school on his behavior — if he was calm or keyed-up before or after lunch. At the end of the week we compared records of what I fed him and the behavior that resulted. We found which foods were causing the problem. I was thankful for his teacher's cooperation

Harris takes his lunch from home and is not allowed to accept food from anyone. If he does, I usually can tell. His behavior gives him away. I usually don't have to worry about him now. He has disciplined himself not to accept food from other children, even when they pressure him. He knows from experience that his body will react negatively. As a result, he might end up losing friends through abnormal behavior that results.

Not everyone can be blessed with a helpful and caring teacher, such as Harris had the year we started. No wonder he wanted the same teacher again the next year! In fact, he almost refused to attend school without him.

First, the teacher was the warm and understanding person I had prayed for. He was easy-going, soft-spoken, gentle. Although his name was Mr. Kennedy, the children called him Mr. K. His creative ideas and patience motivated Harris in positive ways. Harris trusted Mr. K. because he showed that he cared.

Mr. K. encouraged Harris to come to his desk any time and ask how to do his schoolwork. Because of his learning problems, it was hard for Harris to understand and follow simple directions.

Previously, it had been difficult for Harris to ask teachers any questions regarding his schoolwork. He was frightened of teachers because he had been fussed at so much by so many. They would often bark, "You should have been paying attention!" when he had been trying to. Consequently, he merely sat pretending to be doing his work. The D's and F's on his report card proved it.

Then at last! He found Mr. K., a very special teacher who didn't care how many times he asked questions or how much special attention he needed. Mr. K. believed he was there to help the children who needed it most.

Second, Mr. K. painstakingly kept a file of cards, recording each day Harris's behavior and progress on his diet. He wrote lengthy messages on the cards throughout the day.

Third, Mr. K. was a great inspiration. He gave me the faith and encouragement I needed. When I mentioned changing Harris's diet for the better, right away so many people labeled me as a "health fanatic." Instead of being commended, I was ridiculed. But Mr. K. felt sure I could find some answers to our plight through diet. He was a once-in-a-lifetime teacher, there at the right time.

## List All Foods

Following a thorough elimination diet might seem rather strict, but I found through my own encounters (after many blunders) that it is best for the child to forego all offending foods. Then after improvement, introduce the foods back into his diet, one at a time. Then, with the diet diary, try to pinpoint exactly which food gives him an unfavorable reaction. *Don't leave it to memory!* Just be sure and list all foods in the diary. This does not have to be done forever, only until the most troublesome foods are pinpointed.

I made the early mistake of not eliminating all the foods I should have. As a result, I had an extremely tough time trying to trace the culprit foods. My mistakes taught me some new lessons. I should have started from a strict diet, then added questionable foods slowly, watching Harris's reaction as I did.

Now that groundwork has been laid for keeping track of culprit foods, you need to be acquainted with the complicated nature of allergy. Assistance is at hand.

# 10. Food: Friend or Foe

On the Friday before his eighth birthday, Jake and a friend took their baseball bats and smashed every window in their vacationing neighbor's home. When caught at the scene, Jake brazenly denied doing the damage, and placed the sole blame on his friend.

This was the last of a steady series of wrongdoings. Others included lying, cheating, stealing from a nearby supermarket, lighting fires, frequent fights, etc. This last act was the turning point in Jake's life.

Jake was severely hyperactive. His mother, Sharon, had taken him to many specialists before causes of his hyperactive behavior were found.

"We were fortunate to find a physician aware of how undiagnosed food allergies could affect a child's behavioral problems," Sharon explained. "Jake was found to be allergic to almost forty different foods. When these were withdrawn, he became a good-hearted, even-tempered child. His shenanigans decreased."

## Allergies Anyone?

Food allergies are among the most mysterious, frustrating, and confusing ailments. The problem is complex. Symptoms are like a patchwork quilt in their variety and combination. Eating is something most of us do automatically. But to some, even a single bite of the wrong food can cause food allergy symptoms.

I once believed food allergy meant that if I was allergic to a particular food — such as strawberries — I would break out in hives if I ate them. However, food allergies are extremely common and their symptoms can affect all body systems. In short, most allergies are caused by a sensitivity to something eaten, breathed, or touched, and they can show up as behavioral as well as bodily symptoms.

Food allergy can cause a smorgasbord of misery. These symptoms include: anger, anxiety, tremors, mood changes, hives, depression, dizziness, drowsiness, insomnia, fatigue, irritability, nervousness, changes in speech, withdrawal, rapid pulse, hyperactivity, learning disabilities, difficulty in concentrating and remembering, recurring headaches, and just vague complaints of "not feeling well."

In addition to the usual symptoms, food allergy can cause nausea, diarrhea, vomitting, bloating, excessive belching, abdominal pain, flatulence (passing gas), nervous stomach, constipation, and others.

Although respiratory allergies are more likely to be due to inhalants (what is breathed), they may also be caused by foods, resulting in asthma, bronchitis, chronic or seasonal hay fever, sinusitis, and post-nasal drip.[1] And, as any parent of an allergic child can tell you, some can be extremely difficult to identify.

The children most prone? Dr. Smith says, "Blond, blue-eyed kids are the most likely ones to have allergies."[2]

In *Prevention,* Dr. Crook says, "Ninety-four percent of the hyperactive kids I've seen are allergic to foods or food colors of some sort. With an elimination diet, I've found there's a five- or six-to-one chance the behavior can be controlled without drugs."[3]

Gail's son, nine-year old Troy, is a good example. He had asthma from age two.

"He had boundless energy," Gail said, "and I had no idea where the energy came from. Often it was explosive and violent. He would come home from school and start kicking the door. He had punched gaping holes in his bedroom wall and torn off the wallpaper. He was always beating up small children and stealing."

Red dye — in his favorite barbecue-flavored potato chips, Red Hots and cherry flavored soft drinks — turned out to be the culprit.

Allergy can be defined as an overly sensitive reaction to things, which would not occur in the normal person. It is a misguided defensive response by the body's immune system. If bacteria enters the body, it is normal for various cells, antibodies and chemicals to attack them. But if the immune system responds the same way to a harmless invader, it is an allergy.

The first step is to determine what substances set off the allergic reactions. Then one can eliminate or reduce the exposure, depending on the severity of the reaction.

The allergic response to food appears in two forms: either immediate or delayed. In the immediate form, allergic symptoms develop within minutes after eating the culprit food, while delayed symptoms can occur up to several hours later.

Symptoms are affected by many factors, such as the quantity of food eaten, the length of time over which it is consumed, and the number of allergenic foods eaten in combination. All of these may cause a variation in the type, severity or duration of symptoms.

Make a list of your child's main foods — especially favorites — and you will probably find the most frequent causes of food allergy. Allergy-related illness is usually based on exposure, so that the greater the exposure, the greater the likelihood that an allergy will develop to it. Remember, the foods to which your child tends to be allergic to are the ones he eats most often.

Dr. Crook notes in his book *Tracking Down Hidden Food Allergy*: "Hidden food allergy is caused by foods you or your child eat daily, or several times a day. *The person with such an allergy tends to become allergic to his favorite foods.*"[4]

Edna, the mother of a six-year-old daughter said, "Carrie used to gorge herself daily with bread. During the testing, she was found to be allergic to wheat."

## Cyclic Allergy

There are two kinds of food allergies: fixed and cyclic. The latter is most common — ninety-five percent of all food allergies are cyclic.[5]

A cyclic food allergy means that if a child becomes allergic to a particular food, which is then eliminated from his diet, some tolerance is gained for that food. In other words, over time he will lose some of his allergy to it. The result is similar to a heated pan left to cool off.

After he abstains from the food for a period — usually several months — and the food is then reintroduced, an adverse reaction may not occur unless the food again becomes part of his daily diet. But if it does, trouble can start again and cravings for the food can run wild.

This is the importance of the rotation of foods. Referred to as the "Diversified Rotation Diet," it means that a food is eaten not more than once every four days. Slowly a child will build tolerance for that particular food. But if it is eaten more often, the allergy cycle will start again. By not eating the cyclic allergens too frequently, the build-up of toxins that cause severe reactions can be prevented.

I have found, with Harris, that the effect of a particular food will vary on different occasions, with the exception of sugar. In some cases and with some foods, he could eat the food before his system builds up a tolerance. Those foods had to be eliminated from his diet for a longer period before he could begin to develop a tolerance for them.

For instance, cheese was the food Harris found most difficult to give up. It was in his favorites, especially pizza. But my experiments proved that cheese turned him on. An hour after eating a cheese sandwich, Dino became his victim. He chased the dog around the yard pummeling him with his fists.

So I removed cheese for many months. Now, he can eat it once a week with no problem.

## Fixed Allergy

A fixed food allergy is permanent, but fortunately it is less common. This type of food always produces symptoms, and consequently it cannot be reintroduced again in the diet. Even though the child avoids the food for months or years, when he eats it again, he will react.

According to *Dr. Mandell's 5-Day Allergy Relief System*: "It does not matter whether you have eaten the food along with another food, or whether you have only a small amount, you react."[6]

When a child has this type of food allergy, he is usually stuck with it for life. He has no choice other than to avoid the food. Five percent of food-sensitive persons fall into the fixed allergic category.[7]

Lorie's ten-year-old son, Andy, falls into this category. The school officials said he was slightly learning-disabled. Friends said he was just a normal boy. The pediatrician said he was severely hyperactive.

"We were told to start looking for an institution," Lorie said. "Instead, we looked for an allergist. Andy was allergic to milk. No matter how long we left it out of his diet, he still reacted violently upon its reintroduction."

The more commonly consumed foods are the ones which usually cause allergic reactions. Normally, the most common allergenic foods are cow's milk (more than 60% of all food allergies — the number one offender in children), chocolate, wheat, corn, eggs (usually the egg white), citrus, beef, and pork. Sometimes these foods are the most difficult to avoid as they are all widely distributed in the average diet. Some prepared foods contain several of these foods together.

To test a specific food to see if it is a potential allergen — for instance, eggs — Dr. Doris J. Rapp, a Buffalo, New York, allergy specialist and author of two books on the subject, (*Allergies and the Hyperactive Child*, Sovereign Books; *Allergies & Your Family*, Sterling Publishing Co., Inc.) suggests the following. Feed the child the food on Monday and then no more for the next five days. On Sunday morning, give the child the usual amount of that food on an empty stomach. If it is the culprit, exaggerated symptoms should appear within an hour. Wait until this food's symptoms subside — possibly several days — before testing another food.

When the blood sugar fluctuates from allergies or ingestion of sugar or another food that causes reaction, the body tends to go into acidosis (an abnormal increase in the acidity of the body's fluids, due to acid accumulation or bicarbonate depletion). This can have an adverse effect on the body and brain, which, in turn, can be associated with behavioral changes, such as being unruly, uncooperative, or hyperactive.

Many parents have discovered that Alka-Seltzer Gold in the gold packets (sodium and potassium bicarbonate, and ctiric acid — no aspirin) dissolved in a half-glass of water, has helped to lessen the reactions and settle them down.

Dr. Rapp suggests taking a half teaspoon of baking soda in a half glass of water, followed by a full glass of water. A laxative, such as milk of magnesia, also will help terminate the reaction by more rapidly removing the offending food from the intestinal tract.[8]

## Allergic-Addiction Syndrome

Allergy and addiction are closely related. A term has been coined to summarize the clinical observation of this biochemical phenomenon — "Allergic-Addiction Syndrome."

The process works like this: When the allergic person loves a food so much that he feels he must have it daily, and it has a negative allergic effect on him, his body's defense mechanisms swing into action when he eats it. He feels a definite physical and mental boost, a "high," like a drug addict's fix.[9]

As he keeps eating the allergic food, it becomes addictive. He now craves this same food, because he obviously has found he feels so much better if he eats it. He feels he must have the food frequently because he starts feeling bad, experiencing symptoms of withdrawal, if he doesn't.

So if a person actually loves a certain food so much that he must have it every day, he surely has a biochemical need,[10] but most likely it's the very one food he should do without. If the addiction continues long enough, however, his whole immunological system may begin to fall apart. He will then begin having allergic reactions to all types of foods and substances.

In another book by Dr. Crook, *Are You Allergic?* (a must to read!), he explains: "It may surprise you to know, if you have a hidden allergy, you may become 'hooked' or 'addicted' to the food that disagrees with you. So you crave it."[11]

Try to discover those foods your child asks for regularly or sneaks when you're not looking. Although he is not consciously aware of it, his body is sending signals that it needs the food to avoid withdrawal or hangover symptoms, ranging from slight fatigue to severe anxiety, headache, depression, irritability, restlessness, exhaustion, inappropriate behavior, etc. If this sounds like alcoholism, it is — because they are related syndromes.

Look for the foods that make your child jovial or "high." When he comes down from his high, you usually will have to contend with crying, screaming, fighting, depression and temper tantrums.

Ten-year-old Betsy repeatedly asked for chicken, which made her "high." When she came down from her highs she would dive into hysterical, screaming fits. She had a serious food allergy to chicken.

Often a child will show withdrawal symptoms on an elimination diet. He might seem to feel worse the first two or three days. Part of these symptoms might be caused by hunger, or because he craves or is addicted to some of the common foods which have been eliminated, such as milk or sugar.

Food allergy is insidious. For instance, if your child was allergic to poison oak, you would keep him as far away from it as possible. In the case of food allergy, however, the symptoms may be masked, or you may be unaware that the symptoms are being caused by food. (It does seem hard to believe that the child's favorite food could be causing his outbursts of temper, restlessness, depression, diarrhea, earaches, difficulty in concentrating, etc.) Ironically, rather than identifying and avoiding the offending foods, the child may actually gravitate toward them.

A mother of a five-year-old son said his earaches disappeared when milk was removed from his diet.

Does your child's bad behavior improve or disappear when he is ill and is unable to eat anything for several days? This could very well be a clue that he has a hidden food allergy. Other clues to watch are a family history of allergy, low blood sugar, diabetes, alcoholism, mental illness, or obesity.

If an allergic child reacts to one particular food, he may react to other foods in the same botanical family.

Examples: The Nightshade Family — tomato, potato, chili/red/green/bell peppers, eggplant, tobacco.

The Citrus Family — lemon, lime, grapefruit, orange, tangerine, tangelo, citric acid.

The Mustard Family — cabbage, kale, broccoli, cauliflower, brussels sprouts, radish.

The Cashew Family — cashew, mango, pistachio.

An extensive botanical listing of food families can be found in *Coping With Food Allergy,* by Claude A. Frazier, M.D. (Quadrangle/The New York Times Book Co., 1974).

## Types of Testing:

### Skin Tests

The most widely used and most respected allergy test among conventional allergists is the scratch or prick test. According to Doug Kaufmann, a specialist at Physician's Laboratories, Manhattan Beach, California, a small amount of concentrated liquid food extract is placed over a site to be tested — usually the upper portion of the arm or the back. A small scratch or slight prick is placed over the food. Further testing of that food is based on whether the initial scratch leaves suspicious reactions at the test site.[12]

The disadvantages? The test is inconvenient and somewhat painful for the patient. It takes time for the skin to become sensitive and a doctor may have to perform several series of twenty before he is satisfied. Harris's series of twenty, done on his back, were negative. The doctor then moved on to another area of testing.

Kaufmann also says that many allergists question the realiability and accuracy of the scratch test, and that this type of allergy testing may soon become obsolete.[13]

### Provocative Test

A provocative test is performed either by injection or sublingually, by dripping a known amount of food under the tongue, according to Kaufmann.[14]

Using the sublingual testing as an example, a dilute solution is made of each different food and a few drops are placed under the tongue. If this is the offending allergen, within a matter of minutes the child begins having symptoms, their strength depending upon the harmful effects of the toxic food. Then a neutralizing dose of the offending food allergen is placed under the tongue. In a matter of minutes the child will come out of the reaction.

### RAST

Scientists have developed the Radioallergosorbent (RAST) test. Laboratories that do the RAST have a large file of extracts, each representing a particular allergen. The doctor decides which allergens might be responsible and orders a RAST for each one. Harris's doctor, for example, ordered the RAST for milk, eggs, wheat, and legumes. A small sample of the child's blood is drawn and a few drops are added to each of the extracts. A technician tests for positive reaction.

The RAST is complicated and reliable, yet dozens may be required. It is recommended for people with skin diseases so severe that a skin test is impossible.

## Cytotoxic Test

An exciting development now growing in use is the cytotoxic test for detecting food and chemical allergies. According to Kaufmann (executive director of the lab that specializes in cytotoxic food allergy testing), the word cytotoxic is derived from the Greek — "cyto," meaning cell, and "toxic," meaning poisoning effect. "A cytotoxic reaction," he says, "therefore, may simply be described as a poisoning effect on a living cell."[15]

This allergy test involves mixing a small amount of the child's blood with a particular prepared extract of a food that is to be tested, such as egg, corn, wheat, milk, etc. A lab technician examines the blood sample through a microscope, paying close attention to the white blood cells. If the cells react with the tested substance and become damaged or die, that means the child is allergic to that substance. If they remain normal, it means the child tolerates that food well.

A parent who suspects a food allergy and is unable to find the source by the elimination method should see a specialist about trying the other tests. A pediatric allergist — preferably nutritionally oriented —can be most helpful.

Then there is the clinical ecologist. He belongs to a newer breed of doctors who are finding that many physical and mental illnesses are actually allergic reactions to common foods and environmental elements. They specialize in identifying specific food, inhalant, and chemical exposures.

They have developed new methods of food testing, such as the "Diversified Rotation Diet," which may be unknown to the traditional allergist. An illustration of the diet can be found in *Tracking Down Hidden Food Allergy*.

A rotation diet provides a great range and selection of nutritious foods that most of us overlook in our children's limited, addictive menus. Nature intended the body to get all the many nutrients it needs through a wide range of foods.

William H. Philpott, M.D., is a leading proponent of the rotation diet. He says it is our "first and most important weapon in the battle against addictions."[16]

A child can have more than one food allergy. A varied diet will help prevent future allergies, as well as ensuring good nutrition.

As Dr. Smith says, "Allergies can't do everything, but they can do anything."[17] To alleviate the "anything," culprit foods have to be identified and removed, at least temporarily. If reintroduced, the four-day rotation system will give the child's body time to eliminate the substance before having to deal with it again.

An allergy-free child can be a happy child.

Now that the specifics have been established on how to pinpoint more food culprits, get ready to take an exciting adventure into how and where to find natural foods. This will give your child a new beginning in life through food.

# 11. Food for a New Beginning

Kathy referred to her son, Richie, as a "motor-mouth." He never ceased talking. At six years old, Richie constantly got colds and infections. His teacher said he wasn't able to sit quietly and pay attention in class. He frequently had temper tantrums and was forever quarreling with the other children in his classroom.

Kathy was compelled to find some answers. She began reading and investigating. Articles concerning food allergies and food sensitivities kept crossing her path. She made sure Richie's diet was high in protein and totally eliminated the sugar. She then increased his vitamin and mineral supplements.

Her goal was the emergence of a healthy, happy child from an unhealthy, unhappy one. But she knew that, in order to attain this goal, she would have to eliminate other foods, such as white flour products, additives, and, eventually, milk.

Richie is now an exceptionally bright child. He gets along well with his classmates. His once-terrible temper tantrums have disappeared. Kathy says it is a miracle, made possible by a healthy diet. Kathy became aware that what she fed her son affected not only his growth, but also his behavior, emotions, and mental and physical development.

Richie's story is an illustration of the power of a proper diet. Since a child is what he eats, it is super-important to provide his body with the highest-grade fuel. He must enjoy good health if he is to sit still, pay attention, concentrate, learn properly, and be a nice fellow to have around. Besides, the body's defenses against illnesses don't work well if a child is malnourished.

But, you may ask, how do I look for the nutritious foods that will bring about this dramatic change in my child's life?

A new beginning starts in the food store. The difficulty comes in tracking down wholesome foods once we get there. Thus, this chapter — to tell you how and where to track down these foods.

## Inside Facts

You may want to purchase some of the new foods at the health food store, but it isn't always necessary to pay their sometimes higher prices. Cost is always a major factor. Some foods and vitamin and mineral supplements can be found only in a health food store. You may also find better quality there.

Many health-conscious people shop only in health food stores. A lot depends on the character of the health food store. Each embraces different views on nutrition. Not all carry bulk foods or fresh produce. You will have to search to discover one that best suits your needs.

It always pays to shop around for the best quality foods for the lowest prices, whether at the supermarket, health food store, or natural food co-op, which are gaining in popularity. Since the demand has increased, many supermarkets are jumping on the bandwagon and adding health food sections.

The key is to uncover the good foods, wherever they may be.

Health food stores are primarily oriented toward the consumer, emphasizing quality, good taste, wholesomeness, freedom from adulterants, and optimal health. On the other hand, the conventional food stores lean toward benefiting the manufacturer by choosing foods for their long shelf life, mass production, ease of shipment, etc.

## Prevent Boredom

It's time to expand your child's taste buds and take advantage of the many different kinds of foods available. Find new and exciting foods he may never have tried before — what you think he will like. Harris discovered he liked sunflower seeds, which he never had tasted before.

Try not to give your child repetitious menus. Boredom ruins any diet. Kids have more fun when new foods are constantly tried. Have a few surprises now and then. This approach will have to be more successful and gratifying. He will then be more eager to please you.

The best way to teach your child about his new way of eating is to take him to the food store. Let him help pick out the foods he might like to try. He may even suggest foods you thought he would not like. That's what Harris did with pineapple and coconut.

Once a child picks (or cooks, or grows) a certain food, he will want to eat it. If your child is old enough, he soon will be reading food labels himself. Then he will make a game of helping you find different and enticing foods. Get the child involved, and he will be more enthusiastic about his new way of eating.

Ask him to pick the best produce (such as cantaloupe) by smelling it. Help him to notice the difference in the way foods are shaped, their colors and odors. It is good to encourage questions.

If possible, start a vegetable garden and let the child in on it, or let him grow sprouts in the kitchen. He needs to learn that food doesn't automatically grow in cans, but, like his body, needs nurturing.

Once you get the hang of it, shopping is a breeze. You will automatically fly by areas where you once stopped, lingered, and drooled. But now you know those goodies are out! You will learn to stick to the brands you are looking for. You won't be buying whatever strikes your fancy. You will be using fewer convenience items and avoiding junk foods. Since many children react to the lining of some cans, you won't want to load the shopping buggy with canned items. Besides, canned foods usually contain far too much sugar and salt. You can replace them with fresh foods, which are cheaper and tastier.

Fresh fruits and vegetables must fill in for all the missed goodies. Eating more raw vegetables means your family will be getting more nutrients, fiber, and enzymes. Enzymes in raw foods, destroyed by cooking, are needed for proper digestion, absorption, and growth.

Frozen vegetables are preferable to canned, and only unsweetened fruit juices should be purchased.

By following these principles, you will find that more meals will be made from scratch, just as our ancestors did. Consequently, your grocery bill should go down. At first, it might appear to increase as you stock up on new foods. But after the initial shock of replacing staple items, it should swing downward.

It is necessary to recheck the labels at intervals on items you purchase regularly. Manufacturers do change ingredients in their products, but we can change our minds about using those products as the ingredients change.

## Don't Loaf Off

Just because a food is sold in a health food store does not mean it contains the very best of grains — or that it's an all-natural product. For instance, some foods containing unbleached white flour are sold in health food stores.

Although unbleached white flour is a slight improvement over bleached white flour, it is still a far cry from being as good as whole wheat flour. Read the label on breads. If the product reads white flour, enriched flour, or unbleached flour, then it is not good enough for your child. It must be one-hundred percent whole grain flour.

If you bake your own bread, you will know exactly what you're getting. But that isn't always possible. I purchase 100% stone-ground whole-wheat bread at the health food store. Some natural bakeries grind their own flours, using it the same day, so such a bakery would be an ideal source, if you have one locally. Bread at a health food store usually has been shipped from another city and may not be as fresh.

Many whole grain breads are deceiving to the novice natural food shopper. For instance, brown breads sold in supermarkets pass as whole wheat bread, but are not baked with whole wheat or any other whole grain. They are only "wheat" bread — made with bleached white flour, sugar, colorings (caramel or brown), preservatives (to increase shelf life), and labeled to mislead people. The manufacturers are accomplishing their purpose. They capture part of the whole wheat bread market.

If you bake your own bread, you can add extra nutrition with wheat germ, nutritional yeast, and bran (for extra fiber). One of the chief functions of fiber is to add bulk and soften the stool, thus speeding excretion.

Although the flavor is somewhat different, whole grain breads are good when made with blackstrap molasses instead of honey.

Many children consume far too much wheat. Because of this overexposure (in bread, crackers, muffins, cakes, cookies, macaroni, noodles, spaghetti, etc.), many children develop a wheat allergy. They can eat breads made entirely without wheat sold at the health food store. The bread with the best nutrients is a multi-grain loaf with a combination of rye, corn, soy, barley, and wheat.

## The Gooky Monster

I found peanut butter to be cheaper at the flour mill where I purchased my whole grains than it was at the supermarket. Regardless of where you buy nut butters, read the label and make sure they contain no sugar or other additives. Many popular grocery store brands of peanut butter contain lots of both. It's a good idea to make all your own nut and seed butters if you can. Then you will know exactly what you're getting.

Some children do not like peanut butter! I didn't expect to ever see one, but Harris used to hate it. He ate it anyway, to please me. He has now developed a taste for it and it has become one of his most requested foods. Steven, on the other hand, has "peanut butter attacks" morning, noon, and night. It's the one food he feels he can't live without. Peanut butter is a highly-nutritious food. People can develop a taste for previously-disliked foods, as Harris did.

### Perking up Trouble

Many parents of hyperactive children say coffee calms their child, but don't give it to your child. It will start him early on a caffeine habit.

### Eeny, Meeny, Miney, Mo

I am often asked: If a child wants soft drinks, which is better — the sugared or the sugar-free? Healthwise, a child loses either way. If your child or other family members insist on soft drinks, the best ones are uncolored, sugar-free, and caffeine-free, such as Diet 7-Up, Bubble Up, or the lemon limes. This advice comes from a nutritional doctor. It is best to forego them all. Harris usually drinks sparkling mineral water.

### Morsel Tips

There might be times, such as when traveling, that you can't be too choosy about the foods your child eats. You will have to do the best you can, and pray. If he does plunge into bad behavior, your trip may be spoiled. But then, again, maybe you'll hit it lucky.

When eating in restaurants or fast-food places, don't go overboard since you are unable to see what goes on in the kitchen. The plainer the food, the better, such as a hamburger patty, roast beef, baked potato, crisp raw veggies, fresh fruit, or water.

We usually pack Harris's food to take with us. I always carry a jar of peanut butter or other nut butter. My standbys are: Peanuts, nuts (especially almonds), seeds, trail mix, raw vegetable sticks, dried or fresh fruits, and popcorn. Always try to go prepared. Then when his hunger pangs strike, you will be armed with the right remedy.

When we are visiting with friends or relatives, they are almost always eager to prepare something he can eat. I also find people to be impressed with Harris's new attitude and improved behavior. We find that some friends and relatives have had to change to a more natural way of eating because of health problems. Sometimes it's a relief to them that we are eating a more natural way.

No one can enjoy a vacation with an uncontrollable child and his lousy, negative attitude. He ruins everyone else's fun. Therefore, it is important to keep the child in good humor by supplying him with the right grade of fuel for his "gas tank."

Let's face it. It's hard to enjoy ourselves unless our children are happy-go-lucky, agreeable, cooperative, and easily manageable. It won't really seem like vacation if we are forced to take along a Jekyll-Hyde child. But if his behavior has improved, it makes everything more enjoyable, regardless of where we might spend our vacation —even in our own backyard.

## Opt for Simplicity

Don't get discouraged about the time it takes to prepare fancy meals and snacks. You don't have to spend hours preparing foods. Some can be quite simple. In fact, keeping it simple is a good policy. Do the best you can with the time you have. A good time-saver is to make and freeze extra batches of nutritious foods. You will be making your own "convenience" foods, ready-to-eat.

Your own creativity will take over. You will be adapting and fortifying many old favorite recipes by changing and experimenting to create new taste treats that your child will enjoy.

Involve other family members, discussing, understanding, planning, and enjoying the diet transition.

Learn new techniques such as stir-frying, sprouting, blenderizing, and drying. Learn to use non-traditional foods, such as tofu, miso, or tempeh.

Keep in mind that food processing, storing and cooking can easily undermine the best nutritious intentions. Suggestions on how to avoid these common problems can be found in Chapter 22.

## Snackly Rituals

A rule to remember is: Feed your child often — about every two hours. If a child gets desperately hungry, he will eat anything he can get his hands on — usually something he shouldn't have. We are all that way. Our stomachs sometimes overrule us. When we get ravenously hungry, our resistance is zilch and our willpower flies out the window.

Again, always be prepared. I am continually giving Harris a piece of fish or chicken, a shelled, hard-cooked egg, or small sandwich such as tuna with sprouts. Cheese is good if a child doesn't react to it. Some children can tolerate cheese, when they can't tolerate milk. Peanut butter on whole wheat toast, topped with unsweetened applesauce is good.

Raw vegetables are excellent snacks — raw asparagus is great!. Always have something ready that's wholesome and satisfying for that hungry tummy.

Sometimes when a person becomes extremely hungry, he will eat something he doesn't favor. For instance, I have the least-liked vegetables ready for dinner first — or I put out a snack tray filled with raw veggies. Then if anyone is so hungry and feels he can't wait, he has to eat what is ready.

I cannot stress enough the importance of having something wholesome ready to eat at all times. Be prepared!

## Breakfast is Important

If a child is going to perform well in school, breakfast is an important meal. Protein foods, such as eggs instead of cereal, are essential. Proteins will give a child glucose energy slowly, allowing his brain to function properly throughout the morning.

If we nourish our children's brains, they will act accordingly. Just as a car can be tuned up and the fuel tank filled, so can the hyperactive child's behavior be improved by increasing quality of the foods he consumes. His body should be fed with the highest grade of fuel.

Protein or the complex carbohydrates (grains, nuts, seeds, vegetables, and fruits) should be eaten every two to four hours. They tend to nourish the brain more evenly, and also provide fiber.

Refined or processed carbohydrates (white bread, polished rice, bleached white flour products, including spaghetti and macaroni) and the simple carbohydrates (refined sugars, honey, molasses, syrup, etc.) should be avoided.

It's best for the child to eat small amounts of protein foods every few hours rather than eating larger amounts every five or six hours. Since protein foods will keep his blood sugar at a more even level, they will help the child avoid irritability, depression, poor concentration, and sugar cravings.

If the child becomes grouchy after physical activity, his blood sugar could be dropping too low. A snack of high-protein food will bring it up again.

Harris is an example. One Friday afternoon he picked up his Legos immediately following the Flintstones. He was kind, charming, affectionate — the ideal child. He gave me a big bear hug and planted a kiss on my cheek. As he left for the swimming pool in his swimsuit, the words rang out, "I love you, Moomhead!" He was to return by four-thirty so he could go fishing on the coast with Beau.

When Harris returned from swimming, I announced I would be tagging along on the fishing trip. Harris usually begged me to go. This time he was quite the opposite.

He shouted, "I don't want you to go! It's no fun with you along. Stay home!"

I was floored. It was obvious that after three and a half hours of steady swimming, his blood sugar had plummeted. He downed a high-protein snack and within an hour, he was settled. He wrapped his arms around my neck and apologized. He hadn't meant a word he said!

This episode made me more careful to prevent his blood sugar from getting too low.

Keep in mind that the calories a child consumes need to be densely packed with nutrients. Since what he eats has to count more toward meeting his daily requirements, there is less room for "empty calories" — worthless fillers such as sugar and other junk foods.

It's evident that refined, processed foods can't hold a candle to whole, unprocessed, natural foods. Health food snacking is the best way. Its taste will be enjoyed and it will benefit the child's health.

A balance of nutrients must be established, whether it be entirely through food or supplementing the child's diet with vitamins and minerals, which are actually concentrated foods. (Natural vitamins are made from the foods themselves, such as vegetables, grains, fruits, or fish oils). Help is on the way.

# PART III
# Establishing a Balance

# 12. Our Supplement Friends

During a parent-teacher conference with Mr. K., we began discussing Harris's diet.

"Did you get to see Dr. Lendon Smith when he talked here last summer?" he asked.

"No," I answered.

"The school made a tape of his talk. If you would like, I can borrow it for you," he said. "It would be good, though, if you could take Harris to see Dr. Smith. I think he could be a great help to the little guy."

This astounded me. "You mean there's a chance Dr. Smith would see Harris?"

"Oh sure, he takes new patients," he said. "I'll get his phone number and call you later this evening."

It was several months before Dr. Smith could see us. He was visiting schools, giving talks.

Meanwhile, I listened to the school's tapes. I was impressed, especially since I had already learned that diet had a lot to do with behavior.

Dr. Smith was diligently trying to pass this good news on to parents, teachers, and others who work and live with problem children.

He found, in his pediatric practice, a connection between behavioral problems and an inability to properly metabolize refined carbohydrates consumed by these children in large quantities. Blood sugar problems are prevalent among them. He found that marked improvement occurred in a sizable number of cases within three weeks after white sugar (and eventually all sugars), white flour, and processed foods were removed from their diet. He also found that large doses of vitamins B and C, calcium, and magnesium calm hyperactive children.

Harris and I anxiously awaited our appointment.

Our August journey was almost five hundred miles. But I would have traveled to the far end of the earth if it had meant hope for Harris.

It was easy to feel comfortable with Dr. Smith. He was warm, friendly, humorous, thoughtful, understanding, and had a sincere desire to help his little patients. All the many good things I had heard about him were true.

Many hyperactive children, he told us, have trouble with their bodies absorbing vitamins and minerals. Some need abnormally large amounts, which they can't always obtain from their food alone. Harris belonged to this group.

Dr. Smith gave him an injection of vitamin B-complex, and we returned the next morning for another one. Unbelievably, the vitamin shots calmed Harris immediately. If I hadn't seen this phenomenal change for myself, I might not have believed it.

I left Dr. Smith's office inspired and renewed — thankful we had made the journey.

I couldn't muster up the courage, so Beau gave Harris vitamin injections every two to four weeks. We noticed a difference immediately after each shot. A wave of calmness swept over him, like a roaring sea suddenly calmed.

The second phase of *The Natural Way Program* is vitamin and mineral therapy. If you are thinking this is quackery, I can assure you, it's not. My son's well-being and cheerful demeanor attests to that.

This could be one of the most important steps toward helping your child. It does take more detective work though, because finding the right amount of vitamins and minerals can be complex. Not one member of the nutrient team can be left out. It's best to obtain the help of a doctor, a nutritionally-oriented one.

## Missing Links

Hyperactivity is sometimes caused by an imbalance of vitamins and minerals in the body. A lack of certain B vitamins can cause psychological symptoms. Or an excess of certain minerals, such as lead or copper, can cause problems. At times, these imbalances are not necessarily caused by an inadequate diet. Some children merely need a larger than normal amount of some nutrients for proper body functioning.

In other cases, their bodies may be unable to get rid of excesses. Oftentimes, they inherit their body chemistry, or the condition could have developed for other reasons. Whatever the cause, the average adequate diet does not meet their special needs.

Behavioral problems in hyperactive children caused by biochemical or nutritional deficiencies can become psychiatric problems that require therapy if not solved at an early age.

If a child doesn't progress much with oral vitamin supplements, vitamin injections should be investigated. It's quite simple to learn how to give them. They are inexpensive compared to a weekly or monthly visit to a doctor for a shot.

An encouraging study reported in *Biological Psychiatry* suggests that hyperactive children respond more positively to pyridoxine ($B^6$)

than to methylphenidate (Ritalin), the drug most commonly used to control hyperactivity. Because pyridoxine, like methylphenidate, might cause insomnia, it is given to children in the morning. The other B vitamins have also been found to keep children (and adults) awake, so it's best to give them earlier in the day.

When we begin reading about vitamins and minerals, it's easy to see the complications involved in finding the proper amount that should be taken for optimal health. In fact, it seems that in every article we find that each person has a different idea of how much of a certain vitamin or mineral works best.

Throughout my struggles for answers, I learned much by simply asking other people about their experiences. Then I tried some out myself. For instance, I asked my friend, Marge, owner of a health food store, what would help Harris sleep better at night. She said she gave her hyperactive daughter calcium and magnesium at night and they helped her to relax and fall to sleep. I tried it and, sure enough, it worked.

It is good to read articles, books — everything available on nutrition. Subscribe to health magazines if you can afford it. I found many good ideas in these, which helped quench my insatiable need to learn more. They also contain some super nutritional recipes.

## Vitamin Thieves

A child's need for nutrients and how they are utilized will vary from day to day. It depends on his age, weight, lifestyle, eating habits, exercise, mood, environment, illness, stress, and a host of other factors. Each of these influence what nutrients (protein, fat, carbohydrate, vitamins, minerals, water) he needs for proper body functioning.

If the problem is stress — physical, emotional, or mental — the B vitamins, Vitamin C and calcium are being lost. With refined sugar consumption there is loss of B vitamins and magnesium; with caffeine consumption, B vitamins; with heavy exercise, fluid and minerals like sodium and potassium.[1]

The average hyperactive child wolfs down far too much sugar; these children seem to crave abnormal amounts. But sugar robs the body of many badly needed B-complex vitamins. Naturally, they must be replaced. And health always takes longer to reach when a child is behind in his requirements.

## Seek Nutrients

In nutrition, both quality and quantity can change a child's behavior. The child whose diet bulges with junk food doesn't get the vitamins and minerals needed to allow his body to properly burn up what is being eaten. With a more healthful, natural diet, however, along with good vitamin and mineral supplementation, a child should be able to improve greatly. In addition, it will do wonders for his personality and popularity.

Therefore, it's best not to leave him to the catch-as-catch-can type of diet, but to make sure his nutritional needs are fulfilled by planning his meals carefully.

Regardless of what kind of diet a child follows, it is important to choose the foods that give him the highest nutritional value for the lowest calorie contents. We all should be more discriminate eaters, avoiding empty calorie foods. Try looking for the nutritional value in all the foods your child eats. Also, try getting more of the foods rich in protein as well as the ones with a high vitamin and mineral content.

If a child needs a specific vitamin or mineral, it is best to have him eat a particular food high in that nutrient. For example, if he is low in iron, he needs to eat liver or oysters, or another food high in iron.

Although dairy products are our best sources of calcium, many children are sensitive or allergic to them, so other sources need to be found — such as chicken, turkey, canned salmon, tofu, nuts, sesame seeds, wheat germ, and green, leafy vegetables.

## Tailored Rules

Some foods might have a negative reaction on certain children but will be good for others. These might include milk products, eggs, wheat, corn, tomatoes, citrus fruits, and nuts. Although the health professionals endorse and support fundamental "rules" for good nutrition, the rules must be tailored to suit a child's biochemical blueprint.

It might be hard for all of us to eat the right wholesome foods all the time. Some nutritionists suggest doing our best for ninety percent of the time and "goofing off" the other ten percent. This isn't possible for the hyperactive child. He must stick to his diet one hundred percent in order for progress to be made.

Some children are reasonably content with themselves — clear-headed and sensible in how they think, feel, and eat. Unfortunately, Harris isn't this way, unless he sticks to his diet one hundred percent. Strict adherence is the only way for him to be a delightful child.

Not only is a child *what* he eats . . . he also eats as he *feels* and *acts*. His body functions along its health-disease line in relation to what he eats from childhood on. His choice of foods governs his emotional and physical state, how he feels and acts, and the level of stress in his life.

The old adage, you are what you eat, should be modified. In a physical sense, what a child eats, it now seems, is also how he thinks, feels, behaves, and is liked and respected by others.

## Requirements Vary

Some of the recommendations in Appendices B and C will help you arrive at the proper amounts of supplementation for your child. These should be used merely as guidelines. If the child has a serious particular problem, it should be analyzed by a doctor. It is best to check with a nutritionally oriented doctor, if you're lucky enough to find one, before starting any vitamin and mineral regimen.

No one can advise accurately and specifically the amount of nutritional supplements a child or adult should have. We all have individual body chemistries with varying requirements. But some nutritionists do recommend higher than normal doses. Many conditions exist that require higher vitamin and/or mineral doses for effectiveness. For instance, Harris needs high doses of the B-complex vitamins, which help stress-related problems. But this doesn't mean your child will.

Harris also needs large doses of Vitamin C. Here's why: Harris was a sitting duck for various illnesses making the rounds. He was repeatedly ill with colds, flu, ear infections, or bronchitis. His winter months were spent in bed sick with these types of illnesses. They seemed to completely drain his body of its energy, leaving him weak and run-down.

Almost every cold turned into bronchitis, followed by ear infections, requiring excessive amounts of antibiotics.

He had been sickly from birth. We went through many painful visits to specialists, but he never stayed well long. He was always stuck with a bad cold or something more serious. One would no sooner be gone, than another was there to take its place.

Vitamin C (ascorbic acid) finally came to our rescue. It was a blessing from heaven. Nothing has been the same since. I had heard and read repeatedly that Vitamin C is great for fighting colds and infections. But I was stubborn and found this hard to believe. Then from my own experiments with it, I was convinced! It does work wonders! Linda Clark, research writer in the natural health field, says that if she were left on a desert island, Vitamin C is the one nutrient she would choose if she had a single choice.[2]

When Harris went a full year without having a cold, it made a believer out of me. It was the *first* year of his life without a cold. It was the first year he had taken large amounts of Vitamin C. If I had the slightest inkling he might be coming down with something, I immediately increased his Vitamin C.

Harris takes a buffered form of Vitamin C called calcium ascorbate, meaning that the acid of ascorbic acid has been neutralized. Too much acid — of any kind — makes him hyperactive.

It's hard to believe the Recommended Dietary Allowance (RDA) suggests only a paltry 60 mg. daily of this essential vitamin. Linus Pauling, Vitamin C's most fervent advocate, takes 3,000 mg. daily and has done so for many years, during which time he says he has not had a single cold.[3]

The miracles that can be accomplished with Vitamin C are not normally done with minimal doses, but with mega-doses. Stress, such as worry, infection or illness, destroys this important vitamin.

Vitamin C may not actually cure a cold once it has attacked, but it can shorten its duration and lessen the symptoms. It can, however, prevent a cold if *enough* is taken *before* one is overwhelmed with the illness and then tapered off after improvement.

We take 500 mg. of Vitamin C within every one to two hours when we feel like we are coming down with something. Some suggest taking 1,000 mg. every hour.[4] What the body doesn't need is excreted in the urine. One of the few side effects from taking too much is diarrhea. Nevertheless, you should find as I did that Vitamin C will work like a charm. You won't want to be without it again.

It's important to note that to get a child's body back in proper working order after an illness, vitamin and mineral supplementation — especially B-complex and Vitamin C — should be increased, along with a high-protein diet.

Hyperactive children are often hyperactive because of allergies; therefore, Vitamin C might help hyperactivity in some way by altering

Our Supplement Friends 99

the allergic state. It's a must for these children. Almost any child should be able to improve. If his immune system is built up and if the allergens are eliminated, he may not have any more colds, flu, or other infections. Prevention is better than cure!

## How the RDAs Work

Recommended Dietary Allowances are established by the Food and Nutrition Board of the National Academy of Sciences. The RDA for a given nutrient is the amount that should be consumed daily for good health. The allowances are designed to meet the known nutritional needs of nearly all healthy people.

The RDAs are reviewed and reissued every five years. The recommendations are set or changed according to a combination of laboratory findings, statistical samplings, arbitrary judgments and the personal bias of the Food and Nutrition Board members. Not all nutritionists and health advocates agree with the RDAs. Many believe they are extremely low.

For instance, Dr. Smith recommends different daily allowances in his "Prevention Diet" in *Feed Your Kids Right*:[5]

## Vitamins

| Vitamin | Dr. Smith's Minimum RDA |
|---|---|
| A | 5000 - 10,000 units |
| D | 400 - 1000 units |
| C | 100 - 500 mg. |
| B-Complex | |
| $B_1$ | 25 - 50 mg. |
| $B_2$ | 25 - 50 mg. |
| $B_3$ (Niacinamide) | 25 - 50 mg. |
| $B_6$ (Pyridoxine) | 25 - 50 mg. |
| $B_{12}$ (Cobalamin) | 25 - 50 mg. |
| Inositol | 25 mg. |
| Choline | 25 mg. |
| PABA | 25 mg. |
| Pantothenic Acid | 25 mg. |
| Biotin | 250 mcg. |
| Folic Acid | 400 mcg. |

## Minerals

| Mineral | Dr. Smith's Minimum RDA |
|---|---|
| Calcium | 500 - 1000 mg. |
| Magnesium | 250 - 500 mg. |
| Zinc | 15 mg. |
| Iodine | 0.1 mg. |
| Copper | 1.0 mg. |
| Manganese | 5 mg. |

Note: See Appendix B, page 182, for U.S. Government minimum RDAs for vitamins. See Appendix C, page 192, for U.S. Government minimum RDAs for minerals.

Of course, Dr. Smith adds, higher dosages may be needed in dealing with clinical conditions and specific ailments.[6]

I have outlined (appendices B and C) the various kinds of vitamin and mineral supplements that should be taken, along with their RDA requirements. I have listed the function of each one, deficiency symptoms, some of the natural sources to give you ideas on the food sources, and other bits of helpful information.

During my extensive study on foods high in vitamins and minerals, I found the best sources to be: whole grain products, milk products, meat, poultry, fish, liver, eggs, legumes, nutritional yeast, nuts, seeds, fresh fruits and vegetables, especially dark green leafy ones. The nutrients from foods such as these are the ones the body needs for healthy functioning. They should be stressed in *every* child's diet.

## Aiding Absorption

Even though a child's diet is excellent in most respects, the ability of his body to absorb the nutrients in food will ultimately determine the state of his health. Hyperactive children eat a great deal. They sometimes fail to gain weight, and they may have trouble absorbing the nutrients in their foods. This is where enzymes enter the picture.

Without enzymes life would be impossible. Enzymes break down all foods into tiny particles so they can pass through the pores of the small intestine and into the bloodstream. Without this chemical breakdown, no food eaten can be digested and eventually absorbed — meaning that the best food in the world will just lie stagnant, and the body will suffer malnutrition. Meaning also that one is not just what he eats, but what he absorbs of his diet.

This is why the presence and activity of enzymes is necessary for the constant creating of live cells to maintain the organs, nerves, bones, muscles, and glands. Even vitamins or hormones cannot do any work without enzymes.

One category of enzymes is digestive enzymes. One can get supplementary enzymes (besides those which the body manufactures) from raw foods or from supplemental natural enzymes extracted from raw foods. These are enzymes which help out with digestion and make it easier for the body to produce sufficient metabolic enzymes (enzymes which run the body machinery).

There are enzymes to digest fat (called lipase), enzymes to digest protein (known as protease), and an enzyme to digest starch and carbohydrate (called amylase, usually found in the saliva).

Another enzyme category of great importance is the pancreatin enzyme group. It contains many important enzymes such as trypsin, chymotrypsin (as well as the previously mentioned amylase), protease, and lipase. Many hyperactive children improve within only a few days by taking pancreatic enzymes with each meal (not on an empty stomach).

After each meal Harris chews a few papaya enzyme tablets, purchased from the health food store. This has helped his digestion. They contain papaya melon papain and prolase (papaya is famous for aiding digestion), amylase, bromelain, lipase, and cullulase.

## Mealtime Supplement

It's best if a child's supplements are taken with his meals so they can be absorbed, utilized and digested along with his food.

This explanation of vitamins and minerals has been to familiarize you with the range of vital nutrients you and your child will gain when you commit yourselves to a new lifestyle.

Friends like these come in handy. Use them!

# 13. Essential Fatty Acids

Recent research indicates a possible link between hyperactivity and problems with prostaglandins, known in the chemist's shorthand as PGs. PGs play a vital role in regulating the functions of almost all our organs. They seem to be especially important in the brain and have dramatic effects on behavior. Therefore, a lack of PGs could cause severe problems.

PGs are made from vitamin-like substances called "Essential Fatty Acids" (EFAs, Vitamin F). Vegetable oils contain generous amounts; safflower oil, corn oil, soybean oil, peanut oil ... also in sunflower oil. These compounds are similar to the essential amino acids in that they cannot be formed in the body. They must be provided in the diet. Although EFA is in the food, a number of things must happen before it can be converted to PGs, particularly a substance called $PGE_1$, to which much research has been devoted, since $PGE_1$ appears to be especially important in brain functions.

One of the crucial EFAs in the making of PGs is a substance called cis-linoleic acid (cLA). Before cLA can be converted to $PGE_1$ it must be converted to a substance called gamma-linolenic acid (GLA) then to dihomogammalinolenic acid (DGLA) and finally to $PGE_1$.

The Hyperactive Children's Support Group (HCSG) in England, an organization with over seventy branches, has conducted extensive surveys regarding the characteristics of hyperactive children. The results of these and other studies strongly suggest that hyperactive children have deficiencies of EFAs, especially GLA.

HCSG has witnessed dramatic improvements in behavior and function in the preliminary experiments with evening primrose oil, the only substantial natural source of GLA. Some children seem to improve when the oil is rubbed into the skin (the forearm, the thighs and the trunk), instead of taken in oral doses.

Since males need about three times as much EFAs as do females, a lack of EFAs would affect boys more frequently than girls.[1] This could be one reason more boys are affected with hyperactivity than girls. There also is increasing evidence that there may be genetic and sexual differences in the ability to form GLA, with males making less than females, and some males making less than other males.[2]

The EFAs are necessary for normal body defenses against allergies and infections. This could be a reason why hyperactives are more prone to allergies and multiple infections of the ear, nose, and throat.[3]

Lack of EFAs could be why many hyperactives have constant thirst and drink excessive amounts of fluids, including soft drinks.[4] HCSG has evidence which suggests that a lack of the EFAs could be blamed for hyperactive children growing up and turning into alcoholics.

Another indicator of an EFA problem in hyperactive children was uncovered by The New York Institute for Child Development. Many hyperactive children don't absorb simple carbohydrates well. Such problems with absorption mechanisms can occur as a result of an EFA deficiency.

Usually, a simple lack of enough EFA in the diet is unlikely to be a problem, but the EFA must be absorbed into the body. Many hyperactives have problems absorbing food from the intestines. So although enough EFA is in the food they are eating, it may not actually get into the body. The child may also not be getting adequate Vitamin $B_6$ and C and the minerals magnesium and zinc, which are needed in order to convert cLA to $PGE_1$.[5] Studies by the HCSG have shown that more than half of the children involved in their study are deficient in zinc.

Evening primrose oil, a natural seed oil, comes to the rescue. It is not a drug, but a dietary supplement available in health food stores in capsule form. Harris swallowed a capsule after each meal and seemed to exhibit a more pronounced feeling of well-being.

# 14. Hair Can Talk

Although each one of the steps I have mentioned is necessary, it would be hard to say exactly which is the most important. Each step is essential, and these different steps work as a team. Each child might be helped in a different way so it is worth trying all of them.

It's always difficult to forecast how a child's body will react to any step. Some show great improvement, yet others may not be affected at all. But that doesn't mean the step was unnecessary. Everything possible has to be tried to solve the child's problems. Some potential solutions can be ruled out if no benefits have been found. For instance, a particular food might have varying effects on different children, but you won't be able to rule that food out until it has been tried on your child. Nor will you want to rule out the "Hair Analysis Test" until you have tried it.

The hair analysis test for mineral imbalance is rapidly growing in popularity. People are gaining more knowledge about its importance. It can give you many clues to your child's body chemistry, and let you know if all the minerals he is ingesting are being assimilated.

Your doctor can have this test done. Or you can find a form in one of the health magazines to mail in to various laboratories. They normally test up to twenty-one minerals, but this varies with the cost.

Dr. Smith performed the test on Harris. It took about two weeks to receive the results. The test showed him to be extremely low in calcium and magnesium — both calmers, as well as sodium, potassium, iron, manganese, zinc, and chromium. He was high in copper.

I had been giving Harris mineral supplements, but his body wasn't absorbing them. I might as well have been pitching our money into a bonfire. A child's body cannot function properly when there is a severe deficiency of minerals, and deficiencies can arise from problems other than a non-nutritive diet.

Many hyperactive children suffer from a malabsorption or poor digestion of foods. Even though some might be eating intelligently and consuming good mineral supplements, they may still be low (or high) in some minerals. Hair analysis reveals this sort of imbalance.

This test will help you balance the body chemistry. It is far preferable to painful and complicated blood tests, which also may not be as accurate as the hair analysis test.

## How to Test Hair

The hair analysis test is simple. Cut about two tablespoons of hair from the two inches of new hair growth next to the nape of the neck, closest to the scalp. The purpose of taking the hair as close to the skin as possible is that this guarantees the hair growth to be recent and reveals the mineral levels of the past several weeks.

The test form has space for vital statistics, such as age, sex, race, weight, height, hair color, and the type of shampoos or other products used on the hair. The hair sample will be sent to a specially equipped laboratory. Although most laboratories carefully wash and dry the hair, you should cut the sample from clean hair.

The test will give you an accurate check on the child's body mineral levels. Then you will be able to correct any deficiencies or excesses. The test should be done again after ninety days to determine how mineral levels have changed after the mineral supplement regimen.

This test can be an important tool to help produce a calmer, happier and healthier child.

Sometimes children are criticized for their actions. They often can't help it, though, especially if their behavior results from a mineral imbalance. Toxic levels of some minerals poison the enzyme system and inhibit absorption of nutrient minerals.

The hair analysis test can be useful as a diagnostic tool in discovering these imbalances, and can serve as an aid in helping to maintain or regain a child's healthy body. A detoxification program can eliminate the severe symptoms of these minerals once they have been discovered.

## Lead Toxicity

Among the symptoms detected through hair analysis is lead content in the body. Lead poisoning is an insidious, invisible health-destroyer. Since it often works slowly, many people are unaware of it until the damage is done. Lead is all around us —in the air we breathe (despite more unleaded gasoline), the water we drink and the food we eat. Some processed foods are packed in lead-soldered cans. Older house paints constitute another major source of lead.

Lead toxicity cripples a child's capacity to learn. In some, it decreases mental ability, impairs attention span and affects language function and memory. Many children have learning disabilities due to lead toxicity. It has been found that some hyperactive children can actually be taken off drugs after the level of toxic lead has been reduced in their bodies. Studies show that children absorb more lead than any other age group, so finding a method of testing this problem is essential.

## Copper Toxicity

Harmful levels of copper can also be detected through hair analysis. Because the body needs very small amounts of copper in the diet, a child is likely to have problems with too much copper, rather than with too little. Copper toxicity can cause hyperactivity in some children. Drinking water might be a significant source of copper, depending on the hardness of the water and the type of plumbing material used. Copper pipes will raise the concentration of copper in domestic drinking water.

## Conquering the Enemy

Calcium deficiency, one of our greatest problems, is often overlooked.[1] Although the claim is made that our food supply contains an abundance of calcium, this claim is not valid — no more so than the myth that we get everything we need in our daily American diet. Over-cropped soils and refined foods are often responsible.

An undersupply of calcium can cause irritability of the muscles, in the form of cramps or spasms. Most common are leg or foot cramps, but cramps or spasms can occur in almost any muscle. A lack of adequate calcium and magnesium can make a child so irritable that even the most tolerant mother can't contend with him.

Few nutrients can increase good nature and well-being in a home as much as calcium. Without it, tempers flare and irritabilities are constant, but with calcium, peace and serenity return. Calcium and magnesium are nature's own tranquilizers. They work as a team. Their lack can throw a child's body chemistry out of kilter.

In his book, *Foods For Healthy Kids,* Dr. Smith explains,

> We are seeing a fairly high relationship between hyperactivity, low calcium, and low magnesium in the hair, a high incidence of

rhythmical habits, plus a craving for dairy products. As a matter of fact, the more the craving, the more likely the child's hair test to be low in calcium. It is as if they know where the calcium is and consume it, but apparently cannot absorb it.[2]

It is well-nigh impossible to get too much calcium, since calcium is considered to be the hardest of all minerals to assimilate. The type of calcium a person takes is less important than whether or not he is assimilating the calcium.[3]

Some specialists recommend chelated calcium for best absorption, while others insist on calcium lactate, calcium gluconate, oyster shell calcium or others.

Harris had a terrible problem absorbing calcium. I gave him various types of calcium supplements — bone meal, dolomite, oyster shell, calcium lactate, chelated calcium. We pretty well made the rounds. Still, his body wasn't assimilating them.

The fault was not in the calcium but in his system. I knew he could take the "right" calcium recommended for his deficiency — in the correct amounts — until it was coming out his ears and we still would not be getting results.

To ensure calcium's assimilation, a number of guidelines must be followed. Some vitamins and minerals must be supplied, along with the calcium, for full absorption; others inhibit absorption.

| | |
|---|---|
| Vitamin D | Either by getting some daily outdoor sunshine or by supplements. |
| Magnesium | This should always be used together with calcium, in a ratio of about two parts calcium to one part magnesium. |
| Phosphorus | Although this mineral occurs in abundance in our country, too much of it can create a calcium deficiency because it can bind with calcium to the point that when it is excreted, it takes calcium along with it out of the body. |
| Fat | Fat, such as in whole milk, is needed to facilitate calcium assimilation. A low-fat diet may actually decrease calcium absorption. |

Tension and sugar also interfere with calcium assimilation, and a normal flow of bile is needed for calcium assimilation.

In general, Vitamin C, hydrocholoric acid (abbreviated as HCL — can be found at the health food store) and digestive enzymes help minerals like calcium to be absorbed.

From the evidence of Harris's more recent hair analysis test, his calcium level has increased, thanks to a diet adapted according to these guidelines. If your child has similar problems, you should follow these guidelines, too.

In the next section, valuable methods are offered to solve problems encountered in dealing with the common, everyday problems of raising and teaching the hyperactive and/or learning-disabled child. There are effective answers. As you grow and learn with your child, you will find these answers together.

# PART IV
# Coping with an "Impossible" Child

# 15. No One Answer

I am curious by nature. I have to know what makes everything tick. As a result — after many years of doing nothing — I decided to find out why Harris was hyperactive and what I could do about it. Have you, too, ever wondered why your child is hyperactive? I found some surprising answers to this question, and you may too.

Hyperkinesis is a term used to describe a child who behaves in a particular way. It is a complex of symptoms affecting the behavior and lives of a multitude of children. They are severely handicapped by their symptoms during crucial formative years. These children are harder to raise and are more difficult to live with than other children, but no two are alike. Their physical, behavioral, and learning problems are varied.

The term "hyperactive" has become widely used and greatly misunderstood. But attitudes toward the hyperactive child are changing. Children with behavioral problems are being discussed and treated more intelligently. Hyperactive children who have emotional, behavioral, and learning disabilities now are not just labeled "bad."

Hyperactivity is a general term. It can be applied to very different children who happen to share certain patterns of behavior which are caused by many different factors.[1]

Hyperactivity is considered to be a biochemical imbalance in the brain. One of the primary problems associated with the syndrome is an inability to concentrate and focus attention. As a result, The American Psychiatric Association now uses the term "Attention Deficit Disorder" (ADD), replacing the term "Minimal Brain Dysfunction" (MBD) that had been widely used in recent years.

This change in terminology reflects an important shift in how the experts view the syndrome. It was formerly believed that a child with hyperactive behavioral patterns probably had brain damage. But more recent studies do not support that concept, according to Dr. Andrew Skodol of the New York State Psychiatric Institute, New York City.[2]

The words "hyperactivity" and "hyperkinetic" are used interchangeably.[3] The correct medical term is "hyperkinetic syndrome." The prefix "hyper-" means overly, above, more than normal or excessive. The word "kinetic" means motion, energetic or dynamic. Therefore, hyperactivity or hyperkinetic means too much activity or motion.

Seventy-five percent of hyperactive children are blue, green or hazel-eyed. Blue-eyed, blond-haired boys top the list.[4] Hyperactivity is more prevalent in boys than in girls, by a ratio of five to one.[5]

Girls tend to be more orally hyperactive, and boys more physically. Girls may be having just as much trouble with their attention span, but they are not as physically active as boys,[6] and therefore do not experience the symptoms as physically.

Studies estimate that from ten to twenty percent of all school age children are afflicted. The number continues to increase. In fact, it is the most common disorder seen by child psychiatrists.

## Causative Factors

Hyperactivity, unfortunately, is not a simple specific disease resulting from one particular cause. It may be caused by many factors, singly or in combination. Of the numerous causes contributing to hyperactivity, damage to the nervous system due to pregnancy events and difficult births (especially *anoxia,* the lack of oxygen) have usually been blamed. But if hyperactivity could result from damage to the nervous system due to pregnancy events, a difficult birth, or an accident in infancy, then it should appear equally in brown-eyed children and equally in boys and in girls. Other factors must be involved.

A lack of certain vitamins and minerals, or excesses of some minerals, exposure to certain food chemicals, food allergies or food sensitivities can contribute to hyperactivity. Exposure to certain environmental chemicals may also cause problems. A child's emotions and stress can play a role.

Heredity is often a factor, just as heredity plays a role in allergies.[7] A family history of schizophrenia or manic-depressive psychosis could be a factor. Problems in carbohydrate metabolism, leading to obesity, diabetes, and hypoglycemia can contribute to the symptoms. Heavy drinking in families of hyperactive children has been found to be a factor, suggesting a link between tendencies toward alcoholism and hyperactivity. The Chinese claim they have virtually no hyperactive children, and there is little alcoholism among Chinese adults.[8]

Frequently the hyperactive child's mother, father, grandfather, or other relative was hyperactive or had learning difficulties. It has been found that especially the male relatives of hyperactive children were more likely to have had a history of difficulties in childhood that suggested hyperactivity.[9]

You may have realized that there is another hyperactive member of your family, perhaps your spouse. When you begin searching for ways to control your child, you may find that he, too, can be helped with a controlled diet, administered with love.

Parents who themselves suffered from the syndrome are less inclined to wait until their child "grows out of it." Many experts believe that the neglected hyperactive child simply matures into a neglected hyperactive adult.

The findings are consistent: many adults who were hyperactive children are restless, impatient, impulsive, super-energetic, outgoing people, given to snap judgments and outbursts of temper. They probably will succeed in their careers in spite of poor performance in school.[10]

Hyperactivity is more likely to pass from parents to children through genes than through training or some other psychological process.[11] But just because a parent has one child with the disorder, it does not necessarily mean he or she will have another one.

Signs of hyperactivity may be noticeable as early as during pregnancy, as a high degree of fetal movement or excessive kicking. Or it may appear right after birth, as excessive crying or too little, restless sleep. A hyperactive newborn may be in constant motion, kicking or rolling about.

On the other hand, the disorder may not appear until the child starts school and is required to sit still. He starts to fidget and "act up." Neighbors and teachers complain because he is impossible to control.

It may be difficult for the parents to distinguish the behavior of the hyperactive child from that of an overactive one. A child who is merely overactive can be controlled, but a hyperactive child's symptoms often seem overwhelming. It often takes a qualified physician to make the diagnosis. The sooner the child is diagnosed and treated, the better off he will be.

Much research continues into the causes and control of hyperactivity. I believe some day there will be an answer to parents' dilemmas. With my fingers crossed, I hope it's soon! But for now, there is no cure or easy solution to the problems of the hypermotor child. There is only control.

Hyperactivity is not, in itself, the cause of the child's difficult behavioral problems. *Hyperactivity is only a symptom.* It indicates that an undiagnosed something, somewhere in the child's make-up, is amiss — organically or functionally.[12] Some system or organ is not functioning properly. His body signs or symptoms can be read as clues to find out what and why. This is the chief purpose of this book — to help you unmask these clues and lead your child to success.

# 16. Smothering With Drugs

At twelve, John stopped taking his daily doses of Ritalin, the most commonly prescribed drug for hyperactivity. Over the course of the next six months, he became a problem at home and school — in all walks of society. No one could control him.

After two shoplifting charges, several acts of vandalism and a car theft, he landed in Juvenile Court. His future looked bleak. He became suicidal. During his session with a psychiatrist and mental health counselor, he grew agitated and spat at them. He was led, handcuffed and screaming obscenities, back to his cell.

In court, he pleaded guilty. His two shoplifting charges were dismissed as part of a plea bargain.

It was evident to his parents that Ritalin had helped John's hyperactivity and erratic behavior, and that he still needed the drug daily in order to cope within his environment. His problems began when he had stopped taking the drug.

John's attorney, juvenile court caseworkers, state child protective service agents, and the deputy prosecuting attorney all agreed that he needed outside assistance. A specialist was brought in to analyze John's condition. The specialist said he firmly believed that John's problems were related to his diet. He clipped locks of John's hair and sent them to a lab for analysis to determine excess or deficient mineral levels in his body.

Meantime, John was told to use Ritalin daily, at least until his severely *nutrient-deficient* body was built up by a change in his diet. His parents were cautioned on the harmful effects of food additives, junk food and sugar. It was also theorized that John's overexposure in an earlier home to some environmental chemicals had played a part. But Ritalin was their only alternative until John's body showed a positive response to the right diet.

Like John, the uncontrolled, hyperactive child has little chance to succeed in the future. His emotional problems may cause him to run away from home or drop out of school. If he does continue in school, he will have repeated failures. As frustrations build up within him, he may turn to crime, as John did. But through effective and early control, there is a good outlook for his future.

Although his exact future cannot be foretold with any certainty, he will have a much greater chance of survival if he receives needed help soon enough. As a matter of fact, evidence keeps accumulating that hyperactivity is *not* outgrown. It may seem to lessen somewhat, but the underlying causes only breed other and more serious symptoms. It is important to note that hyperactive children are more likely than normal children to become violent adults and fall into a life of crime, according to a new study by Dr. James Morrison of the University of California. So it can be a miserable experience for parents waiting for their child to outgrow it, because that may not happen.

## Advantages of Drug Therapy

Hyperactive children appear to be miserable most of the time. Their irritability and low self-esteem is an essential part of their hyperactivity.

The child can be a constant aggravation, both physically and verbally, to those around him. He needs to find acceptance in society and not to feel so "different" from the other children. No child should have to suffer this way if there is a drug that will help him cope and minimize his problems.

Stimulant drugs might improve the child's basic personality, but the best benefit from drugs is enhancement of the child's ability to do his schoolwork. These drugs are stimulating drugs, which work just the opposite on the hyperactive child as they would on the average child. Amphetamine-type drugs usually speed up the metabolism and make the average child more active and alert. When they are used for the treatment of hyperactivity, however, they produce a reverse effect by actually calming the child. They bring about quick results and make him still, relaxed, attentive, cooperative, less distractible, with improved learning abilities. In a sense they "snow him under."

If a child is placed on a stimulant drug and he settles down, he is definitely hyperactive. Harris's doctor says this is "proof" of hyperactivity. Many parents label their child "hyperactive" when, in fact, he is not hyperactive at all, just more energetic than they think a child should be. For this reason, a doctor likes to have valid "proof." (If a child is overweight, he is probably not hyperactive, but is *hypo*active, a term often used to describe the behavior of a child who is *under*active.)

A child may be merely overactive without being clinically hyperactive. Hyperactivity is believed to be caused by a chemical imbalance in the brain. Overactivity, however, can be the result of many factors, such as the child's basic personality, depression, stress from school or home.

One of the reasons why drug therapy should be defended is based on the theory that hyperactive children have a chemical lack of norepinephrine, a stimulant, in an area of the lower brain, or limbic system. The idea that hyperactivity has a biochemical basis is suggested by the fact that in approximately half the diagnosed cases, some of the most distressing symptoms can be dramatically relieved by giving stimulant drugs.[1] Presumably, stimulant drugs raise the level of norepinephrine, thus correcting the chemical imbalance in the nervous system. There is no solid proof that a chemical imbalance in the brain causes hyperactivity, but the astounding specific changes that the stimulant drugs can bring about make it a strong possibility.[2]

## Seek Control

Unquestionably, the child needs to be helped in any way he can be, whether it is from a program such as the one in this book or drug therapy. A child is often labeled "hyperactive," even though he may do many things a "normal" child ordinarily does. This still is blamed on hyperactivity.

The child needs to feel respected and valuable as a human being. He needs to feel cheerful, pleasant, good-humored, congenial, and kind. He also needs to be an achiever who can be enjoyed by others. He needs to be able to truly give and receive love. Stimulants can help accomplish all these.

Drugs will not "cure" hyperactivity. Drug therapy, however, is sometimes the only rational answer. It would be extremely hard for a parent not to give the hyperactive child a drug when the parent knows that it can accomplish for him what nothing else has been able to. The drug can help him cope with the world around him. When he is calm, he can function more like an average child.

I don't want to influence you either way on whether your child should be placed on drugs. A parent needs to do what he or she thinks is right for the child. Some doctors routinely place a hyperactive child on drugs. I am sure some feel, as I do, on the other hand, that every possibility should be analyzed before using drugs as a final step.

After a parent has tried everything and nothing much works, it might be best if he were placed on one of the drugs such as Benzedrine, Cylert, Dexedrine, Ritalin, etc. The benefits derived from this type of drug far outweigh the disadvantages of their side effects.

Of course, many parents would feel that a doctor is merely practicing quackery if he suggested changing their child's diet and *not* prescribing a drug. They might feel it too much of a hassle to say good riddance to sugar. Again, there are some doctors who recommend that the child be given the drug until the nutritional approach has taken effect. This sounds logical.

As an illustration — Richard's parents heeded a doctor's advice by choosing the diet change instead of drugs.

Richard had been diagnosed hyperactive at age five. The doctor said he would never function normally without a drug. The family had a friend whose child had the same problem and was given the same advice — take Ritalin. When the mother went to another doctor, he said he had stopped using drugs to curb the disorder. He said the same thing could be accomplished by changing the child's diet.

Richard's parents tried the diet too. They proclaimed, "The results were terrific! Our youngster is functioning beautifully both at home and in school. He has no need for Ritalin."

## Drugs Mask

Through effective and early treatment a hyperactive child can grow up to be a productive person who has overcome his handicap. But he needs love and acceptance as an individual so he can become emotionally well-adjusted.

Parents should give great thought to their child's problems and explore thoroughly other methods of treatment before any drug is tried. The drug does nothing to eliminate the cause of the underlying condition. It merely masks the symptom. Giving drugs to change behavior is a big step and one that should be taken only when other, more conservative approaches have been tried and have failed.

If you have tried everything suggested here to improve your child's behavior with no results, and if the nutritional approach (which usually takes three to four weeks) has failed to have much effect, then he may need medical help with drugs.

Hyperactive children may not always be able to help themselves when they do wrong. Although they really want to please their parents, it is just more than their bodies are able to do. They are not capable of controlling themselves.

Harris often remarked that even though he knew "God is watching" he still could not control some of his temperamental actions.

For instance — the time he ventured into a department store to purchase an Atari tape. He had his heart set on the tape after saving his money for a long time. The sales clerk said they were out. He left the store fuming mad. The words shot out, "I'd like to blow her brains out with a bazooka!"

Harris later meekly confessed that he knew God was watching him but that he couldn't control his hasty reactions. He said, "The words just come out. I can't stop them."

## Love is Not Enough

Before our ultimate triumph, although I was on the right road, I had not yet fit all the puzzle pieces together. I was doing everything within my power to control Harris's hyperactivity without resorting to drugs. Still, there are times, regardless of how hard a parent might try, the parent fails. If you don't find the desired help in one direction, then you must continue to search for an answer somewhere else.

I am not saying that no one should be placed on drugs for hyperactivity. They can have a very useful purpose. It is absolutely essential that some children have this type of medication. A good nutritional diet, elimination of food allergies and food sensitivities, along with vitamin and mineral supplementation and a heart full of love, may not be enough. A parent owes it to the child to do what is best for him.

It is my belief that a child should be able to improve or calm down naturally, if at all possible, by methods such as *The Natural Way Program*. Many drugs have side effects, but a "natural" way of dealing with the syndrome does not. And yet, when all else fails, it is in the best interest of the child to try drugs.

Harris had been on the additive-free diet for about six months. Although he had made great improvement, he hadn't progressed quite as well as I had anticipated. He seemed to be at a standstill. We still had some pieces to fit into our puzzle. I wanted desperately to track them down so our puzzle could be solved.

When I heard of a doctor who specialized in behavioral problems only forty-two miles from us, I made an appointment.

I eagerly awaited the day we would see the doctor. I felt that all our troubles would end. (Talk about high expectations!) Our troubles didn't end. The doctor seemed to place his many patients routinely on a drug called Cylert. He said that on this drug Harris would be able to eat more types of foods, such as sweets, junk food and most of the other foods his body could not tolerate before.

This tall, slender, clean-cut, western-dressed doctor appeared skeptical about a relationship between hyperactivity and diet. Silently but wholeheartedly I disagreed with him. I still felt that Harris's body would somehow know that these were foods it could not handle in the normal way.

I was disappointed in what this doctor had to say. I felt angry, frustrated, and cheated because I knew a drug would not cure Harris's hyperactivity. It would only treat the symptom and make it more bearable. I wanted the causes of his problems eliminated.

I didn't realize at the time how desperately some children need drugs in order to make it in this world. I had expected a cure-all for Harris and didn't get it. I then knew I had to continue in my own way with trial and error, to reach the root of his problems. Meantime, I thought that, in all fairness, I would at least give Cylert a good try.

The drugs Harris previously had been placed on worked quite well, except for the many side effects. Cylert was no different. Harris did fabulously well on it — if a parent likes to have the child come home from school and keep silent until bedtime. The parents who believe that a child should be "seen and not heard" would have adored him. He would sit in the rocking chair and rock for hours, or amble outside and swing.

Harris couldn't disagree on anything or be uncooperative because he hardly ever spoke. He refused hardly any food. He was in a zombie-like trance. Harris referred to Cylert as his "be-good pills." They did just that — they made him be good. He was pleasant, agreeable, loving, kind — the perfect child.

Ironically, the very drugs he was afraid of and shunned at school from his peers, he was taking daily, unaware of their content. He trusted me to give him harmless pills. He thought they were just more vitamins!

Frankly, the tranquility I experienced was wonderful and long overdue. I had more free time on my hands than I could recall having in a long time. His demands were no longer thrust upon me daily.

But silence is not always golden. He had the most common side effect symptoms from this drug just as he had with the others — loss of appetite, loss of weight, zombie-like behavior and inability to sleep. At 2 a.m., he would still be wide awake. Other reported side effects, which may have developed if we had kept on using Cylert, are stunted growth and destruction of enzyme processes necessary to metabolize and utilize vitamins and other nutrients.

A child should not receive stimulant drugs until he is of grade school age.[3] They should always be called "medicine" to the child instead of "drugs." Most drugs, such as amphetamines or dextroamphetamines, should be taken at breakfast. They usually take about thirty to forty-five minutes to take effect. The child can be calm when he arrives at school. If the drug makes him too quiet, the dosage should be cut back. I experimented on my own and found that Harris could do well on one-third of the prescribed amount.

Apparently I still had a great deal to learn. The drug loses potency after being taken for a time, so it seems not to work as well after a while. The dosage might have to be increased. It is better to give the drug five days a week and let him do without on weekends and during school vacations,[4] when the child is free from the stress and frustration of school.

Stimulants usually are not habit-forming in children, but teenagers and adults may become addicted to high doses, and ultimately become drug abusers. Therefore, the specialists, as a general rule, usually recommend that the use of stimulants be stopped before the child reaches adolescence.

Before being placed on Cylert, Harris was the typical hyperactive boy. He ate a tremendous amount of food, but burned up so many calories racing his engine that he stayed very thin, with match-stem legs. On Cylert, he was losing weight because he lacked an appetite.

I finally decided: "Enough!" I took him off a drug once more. I preferred having him the old way. At least he talked to me, even if he said things I didn't want to hear.

## Experiments Speak

I found through my experiments that there were three different ways Harris could display his acceptable, praiseworthy behavior:
1. He could take the full dosage of the stimulant drug and continue eating all the foods he wanted.
2. He could take a small amount of the stimulant drug and follow his diet on a more lenient basis, eating some of the foods which normally were taboo.
3. He could adhere completely to his diet, meaning that there was no need for the stimulant drug. He was calm, serene, easy to get

along with. His schoolwork improved. His friends increased. Our compliments increased. He didn't have trouble sleeping and he had a hearty appetite.

This was a natural way of dealing with his syndrome. The results were heartwarming!

You should bury any thoughts you might have about experimenting on your own with this type of drugs. They are powerful chemicals. Although I did so and no harm was done, the experts strongly advise against it. Talk to your child's doctor and let him decide.

If I had not taken Harris off drugs, I might not have searched any further for the various other things that were wrong with him. His health may have deteriorated further.

For instance: his sensitivity to milk and sugar. Milk exclusion did away with stomach aches, faulty vitamin absorption, need for high doses of Vitamin C, faulty calcium absorption, excesses of some minerals like copper, deficiency of others like zinc, anemia, low blood sugar, a thyroid problem, food malabsorption and various other food sensitivities.

All these problems had contributed to his hyperactivity. Because I preferred to find the causes that made Harris need a drug, instead of using the drug itself, I believe I have a healthier, happier child. Although he is not cured, we have learned as a team to master his problem most of the time.

There are still some days when I long for the tranquility I experienced when he was on the drug, such as when he has eaten a forbidden morsel, sometimes unknowingly, and we have to suffer the consequences. But as long as he sticks to his diet one hundred percent, he is able to stay off the drug. He also will have one happy mother!

# 17. Unwind the Roller Coaster

Vivian sat staring out the window on a cool California June day. Tears fell from her eyes. As we chatted, she told me she was mentally and physically exhausted, trying to care for her nine year-old son, PJ.

She said he took up as much time as six children, which is why she hadn't had another child. She found she had no time left to do things she liked to do. She had no time for her husband, Joe.

Vivian has a hyperactive child with epilepsy. Double woes. PJ was given Dilantin. He had not had a seizure in over a year. Still, there were other problems. Vivian was at her wit's end. She feared she could not hold out much longer. Her son was too much for her.

"What else can I do for him?" she questioned with tear-filled eyes.

She had been trying to solve some problems through diet. Progress had been favorable, but slow. Like me, she had expected instant results.

Our short visit left her inspired and motivated. I had traveled a similar rocky road. Upon my suggestion that she search for other factors that could be contributing to PJ's problems, Vivian set out to track them down.

First, she found that stress played a major role. PJ lived in a constantly stressful environment. Vivian and Joe argued repeatedly over their son and how he should be handled. Much of their time was spent in solving problems he created. It became a burden to discipline and control him. Various approaches had been tried, but most were unsuccessful. Vivian and Joe felt totally helpless. Their feelings of helplessness over PJ's condition were reflected in their constant arguments.

Second, PJ had a high-strung schoolteacher with little patience for any of the children. When a different job opening with a pay increase sprang up for Joe in another city, he jumped at the chance. They moved almost immediately. There, PJ was given a patient, caring, sympathetic and good-humored teacher. This made a big difference, not only in his school performance, but in his home life.

Vivian found that other factors began to make a difference. The family had to reschedule their lives. As a result, PJ was in bed earlier each night. With sufficient sleep, he was calmer and easier to cope with.

When Vivian took PJ to a new doctor for a check up, the doctor took a blood test and found him to be anemic. Little by little, the pieces of PJ's puzzle began falling into place. Although his behavioral problems didn't disappear overnight, they gradually began to improve.

## Moving Upstairs

After a little while of eliminating problem foods from your diet, your whole family may begin to feel the strain of this new approach. You have probably needed their constant help along the way. You may have learned by now that much can be done to help alleviate some of the emotional problems in the home of the hyperactive child. Possibly other family members have learned how to deal with and understand problems that plague the child.

You probably know what foods are best for your child's individual needs and what foods he should not be allowed to eat. Hopefully, the whole family has improved by being less sick and more cheerful. Some hyperactive children may have other factors contributing to their problems. The best thing to do is to check every single possibility.

As you know, there are many diverse things such as nutrition, body chemistry, allergy and others that might be factors. It would be nice if I could give you the name of one specific doctor who specializes in all the aspects of your child's many problems, but I cannot. It would be false hope to think that one specific doctor could solve all the problems. There are many factors that might be contributing to your child's hyperactivity.

There are specialists available to help your child in all these areas. You, as a parent, will be the coordinator of all these specialists. You follow their advice and determine what works for your particular child. This carries a load of responsibility, but the prognosis is encouraging.

You may run into a doctor not experienced with the necessary treatment program described here. Most doctors are trained primarily in the use of drugs and surgery, and have little or no training in nutrition. If a doctor can see the success you have had so far, he might be willing to work with you. If not, perhaps he can refer you to someone who can.

Perhaps you will be more fortunate than we are in some respects. We live in a small mountain town. We have to travel a great distance, over many winding roads to visit our family doctor. We had to travel even further to visit a specialist — many miles, in fact, to visit various specialists. But I never gave up hope. I did, however, find it surprising that most doctors didn't inquire about his eating habits, although the word "hyperactivity" springs up all over the country in connection with diet.

## Seeking Help

Before beginning a regimen to treat hyperactivity, all health problems should be ruled out — low thyroid, anemia, or anything of that nature. A five-hour glucose tolerance test will show if your child has a blood sugar problem. Even pinworms should be ruled out, since they can make a child highly irritable and restless. Other tests might be indicated, depending on symptoms.

It is best to search for a doctor who understands this type problem. He will be more sympathetic with the troubles you are experiencing.

Unless you find a nutritionally oriented doctor, he may be skeptical, appear to be hostile or even amused at the theory that diet might affect behavior. Instead, he may play the "blame-game" by placing the blame on *your* nerves or lifestyle. For instance, "The mother is nervous, so the child is nervous," or "He's spoiled."

A *pediatrician* or your *family doctor* is usually the first person consulted. He is most familiar with your family.

Every child should have a physical examination at least once a year. At that time the doctor can rule out the possibility that his problems are being caused by some physical ailment or defect affecting his behavior. He can make referrals to specialists, and he has the experience to recognize if the child's behavior differs from that of other children his age. Often a family doctor might be in a better position to judge the child's behavior than the parents.

A doctor knowledgeable and willing to take his time can really be a tremendous help. Some doctors are not much for discussing hyperactivity. Most are better at diagnosing and treating physical ailments than psychological ones. If you feel your doctor doesn't try to understand, or that he can't take the time to help, seek another doctor.

If the doctor refers your child to some other specialist, ask him why. Don't feel embarrassed about asking the cost. Be sure to ask all questions in your mind. Speak up! Doctors are usually more than willing to answer questions.

Various specialists may be recommended, depending on the type of problems your child displays.

A *neurologist* specializes in structure and diseases of the nervous system. He will usually check the eyes, ears and sense of touch. He may ask the child to perform a variety of simple motions — raising eyebrows, winking, walking a straight line, standing on one foot, touching his finger to his nose, holding his arms out in front, etc. He will check the child's reflexes by tapping him with a rubber hammer. He may perform an electroencephalogram (EEG).

An *educational consultant,* also called an educational therapist, can help a child with problems in school. He holds an advanced degree in education — the process of training and developing the mind and character. He is especially knowledgeable about special education, and can make referrals to other specialists.

A *psychiatrist* is one who graduates from medical school and then goes on to specialize in psychological medicine. He has had medical training as well as education in mental illness. He is equipped to recognize the physical aspects of emotional difficulties. Many psychiatrists specialize in children.

At one time many felt ashamed about seeing a psychiatrist, believing people would think of them as being "crazy," but it is more widely accepted today. He can be a great source of help to the child and the parents. He can also advise parents on how to best deal with their child's troublesome behavior.

A *psychologist* is one who has an advanced degree in psychology, the scientific study of human behavior — actions, traits, attitude, thoughts, and mental state. Some have been trained specifically to work with children. His key role in the treatment of a hyperactive child is to assess the child's intellectual capabilities and handicaps and to observe his behavioral style.

*Psychotherapy* is a broad term covering any kind of help aiming to alleviate emotional difficulties. It is the treatment of mental disorders through communication, including suggestions, counseling, and psychoanalysis.

A therapist usually attempts to relieve pent-up feelings of anger, frustration and fear and keep one from functioning at one's best. Psychotherapy is usually more valuable for the parents than for the child, because of the problems they face in raising a difficult child.

*Counseling* generally implies the offering of practical advice to deal with specific situations. It can be an important element of psychotherapy. The type most helpful to the parents of a hyperactive child is counseling on a day-to-day basis, rather than just weekly or monthly. It gives one the chance to talk about his or her problems with a friendly and sympathetic person. He can be reassuring, as well as a great source of understanding.

A speech problem could be a hearing problem. Failure to pay attention or follow directions may result from not hearing normally. If the child's speech development is slow; if he has a marked speech impediment, or if you suspect a hearing defect, he should be taken to a *speech and hearing specialist*. He can evaluate the child's hearing and language functions and carry out corrective therapy.

An *ophthalmologist* is a medical doctor (M.D.) who specializes in the structure, function and diseases of the eye.

An *optometrist* is a specialist (not an M.D.) who measures the powers of sight and tests the eyes. He prescribes glasses to correct any defects.

## Bedwetting

Bedwetting can sometimes appear to be more of a problem to the parents than for the child himself. Until it becomes a social problem for the child, there may be little need for concern.

The cause of this annoying problem is usually unknown in the majority of cases. Genetic factors are often the most common causes. Adults who wet the bed when they were children are more likely to have children who do so.

Bedwetting affects more boys than girls. Most children outgrow the habit without any special help from their parents. Harris was nine before he stopped completely.

Many children wet the bed because of fluid intake after four or five o'clock p.m. Milk allergy can be a factor. For reasons specialists do not yet understand, bedwetting is quite commonly associated with hyperactivity.

A good attitude toward bedwetting: If it is not a big problem for the child then it shouldn't be for his parents.

A child who wets frequently during the day and has poor control should be seen by a *urologist*.

## Land of Nod

A specific time needs to be set for the child's bedtime so he will always know when to expect it. If he wakes up easily the next morning, then you know he's getting enough sleep. Take into consideration his age and his individual needs for sleep. Some children need more, some less. Harris needs a great deal or he becomes grouchy. His friends manage with two hours less.

Sleep is that special time the body devotes to normal repair and maintenance to keep the child in the best of health. It refreshes and revitalizes him. An adequate amount is essential.

Many hyperactive children have trouble going to sleep. Many awaken during the night. Some sleep lightly, restlessly twisting and turning all night. Many are late-to-bed and early-to-rise. The same pattern does not fit every hyperactive child. But with a more natural and nutritional approach, his sleep patterns should improve.

When asked why it takes a hyperactive child longer to go to sleep, the authors of *Your Hyperactive Child* reply that "his battery is still charged" — his brain is still working overtime.[1]

They also say that his control mechanism doesn't lend itself to spontaneous relaxation, and that the reason he doesn't sleep through the night is because his brain is constantly stimulated. The emotional problems that present themselves during the day must be expressed and released. This usually occurs during his sleep, causing him to waken often.

## Hypothyroidism

Many children have symptoms of hypothyroidism (low thyroid), such as fatigue, depression, over-sensitivity to cold (usually cold hands and feet), high susceptibility to colds and respiratory ailments, drowsiness, constipation, skin disorders, hair loss, mental sluggishness, poor memory/concentration/learning, hyperactivity, headaches, or slow heart rate. Since the thyroid hormone is involved in the metabolism of every cell in the body, a thyroid work-up should be a part of the hyperactive child's examination.

Probably the foremost leading expert on thyroid function is Broda Barnes, M.D., physician and thyroid physiologist. He has devoted much of his career to the study of thyroid disorders. He says hyperactive children respond quite well to thyroid administration if they have a low basal temperature.

Since many hyperactive children are at the low end of the normal range for thyroid function, some doctors treat them with thyroid hormone.[2] Although we often think of stimulants as calming the high-strung, hyperactive child, we fail to think of a thyroid hormone as doing so. But Harris responded remarkably well to it.

Harris always had plenty of energy to run, jump, and play, but when it came time to do chores — like stacking wood — he complained, "I don't feel like it. I'm too tired."

We began to think we just had a lazy son on our hands. Then shortly after taking thyroid hormone, he no longer complained of fatigue or not feeling well. When wood stacking time came, he eagerly stacked, singing all the while. Another benefit was that he was calmer than ever!

There is a no-cost method by which anyone can make the test to see if the thyroid gland is functioning adequately. When the child wakes in the morning, shake a thermometer down and place it snugly under his armpit for about five minutes *before* he gets up. If the temperature is 97.6° or below for several days, it usually indicates that the thyroid gland is under-active.[3] Normal temperature range is 97.8° to 98.2°.

Temperature taken under the armpit is usually more accurate than from the mouth, because colds, sinusitis, and other infections affect mouth temperature. If the thyroid gland is not functioning adequately, thyroid hormone replacement may be necessary.

## Stress

Stress is a word used to describe the way the body copes with difficult situations. Stress is anything that puts an extra load on the body. The body can't differentiate between one kind of threat and another one.

Hyperactive children are especially vulnerable to the effects of stress. A physically and emotionally, healthy environment is crucial to the successful management of stress.

Some of the familiar symptoms of stress are: sullenness, anger, short temper, hostility, depression, phobias, headaches, allergies, tension, and stomachaches.

Many things can place an extra load on the child's body, resulting in a stressful situation. Some are: faulty nutrition, pain, infections, emotional upsets, diarrhea, anxiety, lack of sleep, exposure to heat or cold, taking drugs, crying spells, inability to concentrate, destructive behavior, and others. To the hyperactive child, even simple things put an extra load on his system — brushing his teeth, going to the bathroom, eating, playing, getting dressed for school, or answering the telephone. The more stress on a child, the more symptoms occur. His symptoms may be worse during school days, which means that there are more anxiety-provoking situations in school than at home.

Stress can make some children more susceptible to disease. Stress has been blamed for a variety of gastrointestinal ailments. Harris had this type of problem for a year. He was miserable, with constant symptoms of nausea, fever, vomiting, and diarrhea. After blood tests and X-rays the diagnosis was "irritable bowel syndrome." The doctor prescribed medication to relieve the symptoms, but we had to work as well to reduce the stressful elements of his life.

The child should be placed with a tolerant teacher. Some children act up with one type of teacher more than another. The wrong teacher can place stress on him. Try to do everything possible so the child has less stressful situations in school. An understanding teacher is one of the best allies a parent can have.

The family should adhere to a normal routine, so he will know exactly what to expect. Routine is an important part in the life of a hyperactive child. He will be more tense and nervous when there is no schedule. He needs to follow the same routine from day to day: getting up and going to bed at the same time, sitting at the same place at the table, being served his meals at the same time, sitting in the same seat at school each day.

It is best to prepare the child ahead of time for a change in routine. Any uncertainty about what is going on in his life places him under severe stress. He will do much better in a non-stressful atmosphere.

One way for a child to relieve tension is with action, such as hitting a pillow, a punching bag, or anything else that is suitable.

Harris rocks in a rocking chair as a tension-reliever. As a baby, he rocked and shook his crib so hard it would nearly fall apart. As he grew older, when he became angry or upset, he darted for the swing. He had to be moving all the time.

It helps for the child to get involved in a hobby to relieve his stress. Basketball, football, soccer, table tennis, volleyball, and swimming are all good, as is playing a musical instrument (especially drums; at one time Harris played more than two hours a day!) He needs a variety of activities as outlets for his energy. It is wise, however, to avoid highly competitive sports, because they create more stress.

## Another Link

Each family has its share of illnesses, but an illness can be devastating to a hyperactive child, totally exhausting his body. Evidence indicates behavioral problems, allergies, and infections are prone to recur in the same children. Nervous children are likely to have a higher rate of ulcers, irritable bowels, tiredness, and anxiety.

Allergy should be suspected when the child is often ill. If allergies are controlled, the child may have less illness. Allergic children are more prone to ear, respiratory and intestinal infections. They more often require more antibiotics for asthma, bronchitis, and fevers.

A child who is often ill can't help but feel tired and irritable. He will have no appetite and be unable to sleep. It will take more time for such a child to recuperate.

## Behavior Therapy

There is a therapy technique called "behavior modification," effective on some children with disruptive behavior. Children like rewards and will usually work for one. A parent might offer a reward — money, a toy, a favorite TV program, or more of the parent's time — for an improvement in his child's behavior.

The reward could be given for not moving so much, for not arguing, not saying a cross word or not screaming. These rewards must be *directly related* to the bad behavior. The system is an excellent motivator for him to do his best. Later, he can be rewarded with merely good words or lavish praise.

Marty is an example. Every Sunday morning in church, he squirmed throughout the service. The whole bench in the old church building squeaked and slid around. It was embarrassing for his family. "If you don't stop it, I'm going to . . ." didn't work. What could be done?

Marty's parents offered him a reward for being still. If he would try his best to remain still throughout the service he would be allowed to stay up thirty minutes later that night to watch his favorite TV show. Later, when the show was taken off the air, Marty received only words of praise. It worked.

All the pieces of your child's biochemical idiosyncrasies may not fall into place automatically in a short time. Sometimes it takes a while, as in PJ's case. In time, though, you should see favorable results, and you can begin to feel optimistic about your child's future. Someday — it may come as a pleasant surprise to you — he will draw compliments instead of blame.

# 18. Characterstic Pattern

"At least several times a week children are brought to my office who appear as if stamped out of the same mold," says Dr. Smith.[1]

Tommy, a hyperactive ten year-old boy, fair and blue-eyed, had a thin puny body, a long thin narrow face, with dark circles under his eyes, a crowded dental arch and buck teeth. He fit the pattern. He had repeated ear and bronchial infections and was ticklish, restless, and unable to sleep through the night.

Tommy had a Jekyll-and-Hyde personality. At one time he would be calm, bright, cheerful, thoughtful, agreeable, and cooperative. Then he would become horrid, hateful, crying, screaming, unhappy, disagreeable, and intolerable.

Tommy was also fond of foods with sugar and refined flour. He gulped down junk foods. He had more than his share of cavities.

When Tommy began fourth grade, his problems became full-blown. He was disruptive in the classroom and disturbed the other children. His attention span was short. His teacher found him unteachable. He was always fighting with other children.

When his mother caught him trying to bash his best friend's head in with a stick, she took him to a doctor. Tommy was given Ritalin. His parents never considered changing his diet. Although the drug helped calm him, his infections continued.

Each time Tommy went for a check-up, the doctor said, "He'll outgrow it." Tommy is now sixteen. Most of his problems still plague him. He is a typical hyperactive child, and the typical advice was given to his parents. They had no understanding of his disorder.

Before we can fully understand what to do about hyperactive children, we must have a more precise picture of the problems and how the syndrome of hyperactivity affects behavioral patterns. Then we will be able to help the child. In addition, we can avoid development of other emotional problems in our children and ourselves.

The term "hyperactive" describes a child who is overactive, restless, easily frustrated, aggressive, irritable, distractible, impatient, impulsive, immature, unpredictable, compulsive, easily excitable, and a non-stop talker. He has a high-strung temperament, won't take no for an answer, is hard to handle, lacks self-control, is unaccepted by friends, has no fear of danger, and is constantly on the go. He also has a short attention span and usually has trouble in school.

These are only a few common characteristics of hyperkinetic children. They will not fit every child, because there are many degrees of hyperactivity. Severity of the symptoms varies. These should be a clue as to what the child is up against. His body is signaling for *help*!

It is important to realize that not all hyperactive children are learning disabled and that not all learning disabled children are hyperactive.

Parents of a hyperactive child are often confused by the inconsistency of his behavior. At times his hyperactivity might seem to be quite severe, while at other times it almost seems to disappear. When it is worse, it is usually associated with emotional stress, although the restlessness, distractibility, and other traits prevail all the time. Intensity of the overall problem varies, but displays itself during stressful periods, when the child is faced with a new experience, pleasant or unpleasant.

Parents cannot take this child anywhere without creating an unpleasant or conspicuous scene. Although he might appear to be normal to a family with a high activity level, he might be just an unpleasant nuisance to a calm and quiet family. Some parents might view their child as merely being overactive, while friends or relatives might consider his behavior bizarre.

For example, Tim's family had a high activity level and consequently thought nothing of Tim being overactive. However, the family's friends, relatives and Tim's schoolteacher saw him in a different light. When a close friend suggested that Tim be checked by a doctor, Tim's mother took the advice. The friend's hunch was on target.

The hyperactive child's unceasing, restless motion and his emotional swings are a strain on his parents. They create a tense environment in the home. There is usually much screaming, fighting, and tears. Coping with him can be more than his parents can tolerate. He doesn't always respond to discipline. He has little or no control over his behavior.

Parents are often hurt to see the child they love so much becoming unpopular and despised by his peers. They know he can be a loving, affectionate and good-natured child. Basically, he is friendly and outgoing. Everybody may like him... at times. If he were only able to sustain good behavior we would all be much happier.

Take for instance, seven year-old Robert. When a new boy comes to school, Robert is always the first to greet him with a smile. He makes the newcomer feel at ease with his friendly personality. At recess, Robert spends all his time with the newcomer explaining the daily routines. Robert's charm is turned on full blast. He finally has a friend!

By the newcomer's second day, Robert has already shown his true personality. A fist fight starts. Then Robert begins calling the boy names during the day. He knocks the boy's books to the floor (accidentally, of course!). Robert and his short-term new friend become bitter enemies.

Robert can be good-natured, but only for a limited time. He is unpopular with his peers. They try to stay clear of him and his explosive temper. At home, it's no different. Friends never come to his house to play. When he calls, they make excuses. They go to Johnny's house down the street.

Robert is hurt because no one likes him. His parents are hurt, too. They know how pleasant Robert can be — sometimes.

## School: Worst Affliction

The child unable to learn is unteachable, or at least he cannot be taught by the usual group methods in the average classroom setting. Therefore, the hyperactive child usually doesn't do too well in school. School is his worst affliction. He will have both learning and social problems.

He has trouble with his schoolwork because he can't concentrate. He has the ability to learn the work but is unable to do it. He fails tests, loses books or work, or forgets to do his homework. He also will guess wildly at answers rather than try to figure them out. Because their nervous systems are so sensitive, many hyperactive children are unable to work at full potential, although they may have perfectly normal, or even superior, intelligence.[2]

He usually has a desk close to the teacher's, not always by choice. He does seem to pay closer attention there. The teacher also will find it easier to pay closer attention to him here where he won't be so easily distracted by the other children.

The child usually has trouble because the teacher often becomes annoyed with his disruptions of the class. The teacher may grow tired of his blurting out the answers to questions intended for other children, or his interrupting the teacher's questions to ask questions of his own.

Fatigue and stress often build up in the child. Then it is difficult for any teacher to cope with him. Some teachers may not recognize that the child has medical problems and may regard him as a troublemaker, hard to get along with.

The teacher may punish him constantly for his bad behavior. This will cause his poor self-image to crumble more, and aggravate his condition. He will then begin to view school as a threat, and it will become a scary and painful experience for him.

The child is confused by group activity. He will have trouble because of the many distractions. It is much more difficult to maintain the structure and discipline he needs in a group. Smaller groups work better for him. He will then be more likely to advance at his own rate of development. He would do much better on a one-to-one basis with his teacher, but that is not always possible.

An overly energetic, motor-driven, difficult child who is hard to get along with is a prime prospect for school and home problems. If he develops doubts about his competence, depression sets in. He is nervous and afraid. He has potential if he could only apply himself, but success in school requires a great deal of conformity.

Teachers normally don't have the time or energy to give individual attention to a hyperactive child. A crucial factor in how a child feels about his schoolwork depends on the disposition of his teacher.

Hyperactive boys usually respond better to a male teacher in their classroom. Male teachers are more likely to encourage self-assertion on the part of their students. Harris fared much better with male teachers, although I had been apprehensive about his having one.

The child's teacher may be one of the first to identify his problems. When a hyperactive child is recognized, it is good for parents to approach the teacher and ask for advice on how he can be helped.

Everyone has a fear of failure — of not measuring up. But not like this child. He resents his inability to learn. He blows his top when frustrated and constantly lashes out in anger. He overreacts in any situation, feeling insecure and inadequate. His defiant behavior often is the result of the anxiety in a stressful situation.

If your child is severely hyperactive like Harris, his condition will grow worse in a large-group situation. This may have disastrous effects, by creating further episodes of failure. When a child does poorly in school, he is likely to develop a bad attitude that will keep him from doing better. He feels more adequate when he proves to himself that he can do well in school.

Just because a child has problems in school and elsewhere doesn't mean he will not do well in life. A child needs reassurance of this. Harris worries about it. Even children are able to understand the difference between school situations and other life situations when they are patiently explained.

## Recognize Accomplishments

The child's accomplishments must be recognized. We must remember that he has worked so much harder for them than the average child. We need to let him know we recognize the effort he makes in doing a particular thing. We must *never* take his achievements for granted without comment. He needs those good remarks.

A child has a sense of accomplishment when he does satisfactory schoolwork. When a child brings home samples of his schoolwork, parents should be quick to show an interest. Offer him encouragement. Show less interest in the grades he makes, but more in the effort he puts forth in trying to finish his work.

Place emphasis on his accomplishments and improvements, rather than on his failures. Then he will be more eager than ever to do better the next time. If *he* feels he has done a good job, even though he received a low grade — offer more encouragement. Act proud of him. He deserves it.

For example, when Harris was in fourth grade, he had studied for an important test for two weeks. The day he received his grade, he whirled into the driveway on his bicycle. He jumped off and bounced eagerly into the house with his school paper crumbled in his hand. His hair was rumpled. He was out of breath. His face beamed with happiness. He shoved the paper in my hand.

Excitedly, he burst out with "Look Mom! Look at my grade! I made a 'C'!"

I looked the paper over. Written brightly across the top in red was a "C" grade. Harris was as tickled as if he had made an "A." *He* felt he had done a good job. That's what counts. I was proud of him for the effort he put forth. I knew he had worked so much harder than the average child for his accomplishment. He was still beaming over the "C" grade at the end of the week.

Sometimes hyperactive children benefit from starting school a bit later in life. A child should not start school until he is "school-ready." If parents are unsure if the time has come, it is better to wait another year. If he is younger than his classmates, he will have a tough time competing. When he is truly ready, he will be able to do more satisfactory schoolwork. The praise that follows will boost his self-esteem. He will *want* to work harder, thus will learn more rapidly.

## School Phobia

A great number of hyperactive children have a persistent, irrational fear of school, called *school phobia*. The child might develop imaginary symptoms — headache, stomachache, or sore throat — to avoid school. This is his way of escaping.

Once a child has fallen into the habit of avoiding school through early-morning symptoms, his school phobia may be difficult to overcome. He needs to be encouraged to return to school and to overcome this fear.

Many of these children are reluctant to return to school after the holidays. If no tangible reason can be found, school phobia could be the problem.

If a child is unhappy or unsuccessful in school, he doesn't have much choice but to stay in the same situation from day to day. Even though he does poorly, he still has to continue back. This could be one reason why hyperactive children are absent from school more than average children. The child may be mad at the world because he feels he is trapped and can do nothing about it.

If a child has more trouble at home with his family than at school, he may not be the typical hyperactive child. He may have emotional problems.[3] The typical hyperactive child has more problems when or where there are numerous distractions, such as in a full classroom.

A significant factor in a child's attitude toward learning and his ability to learn is the home environment. He is more likely to do well in school if his home environment is stimulating, if learning is respected and valued and if parents take an active interest in his education.

## Short Attention Span

The most troublesome characteristic of hyperactivity is a short attention span, or distractibility. The hyperactive child needs activities that require change and movement. He is unable to sit quietly. He cannot watch his favorite TV program without wiggling or moving.

In school, he is easily distracted when performing a task. His ability to concentrate disappears. He is unable to finish his work. He struggles unsuccessfully with tasks that require sitting for long periods.

His mind wanders easily, even while being told what to do or not to do. When he begins taking directions, he tries hard to listen, but "tunes out" after the first few words.

Due to his short attention span, he disrupts the classroom. He is unable to stay in his seat for long. He has to be up and about the room. He is constantly active, so he will absorb less information and do less work. He may appear to have a normal attention span at home, but he will go to pieces when there are many children around.

His short attention span interferes with absorption of information. His distractibility makes it unlikely that he will finish his work. As a result, he is unable to keep up with the rest of his class.

The hyperactive child has a poor memory. He may answer the same question correctly one day and incorrectly the next day. He may also have poor reading and writing skills. The resulting frustration aggravates his social adjustment.

He is sometimes unable to repeat simple tasks that he has done before. He may have actually forgotten the method for solving that particular problem.

The hyperactive child has difficulty in concentrating if there are distractions, small movements, noises, or other stimulations. These cause him to be confused and he gives up. Eventually he develops a negative attitude toward problem solving, which brings additional frustration.

Since he can't always control his impulses, he will not always do as he is told. He is unable to follow instructions unless they are repeated in very simple terms. He is too busy going in many different, confusing directions. To add fuel to the fire, most teachers are more ready to discipline and find fault than try to accept the situation and work with him.

Although he is hyperactive, he is expected to "sit still, apply yourself, learn and achieve" — which is asking more than he can give. This child can and will learn, but conditions must be perfect and everything in place for him to function. There can be no disturbance or stress while he is striving to achieve.

In fourth grade, Harris's teacher found it next to impossible for him to take directions. The teacher would have Harris look him directly in the eyes, get his total attention and then proceed to tell him precisely what to do. The teacher suggested I do likewise. I did so, with good results.

It helps to slowly repeat questions or answers in simple, exact phrases he can understand. Try not to confuse him. He already has a problem organizing thought sequences. Try not to be impatient when the questions or answers have to be repeated. It is often a hardship for him to understand and carry out instructions.

Sometimes, when I give Harris instructions, he says, "Mom, tell me *slowly* so I can understand."

When Harris started on his homework, I would explain it and then help him. I got frustrated myself. Sometimes I felt like blurting out the correct answers. It often took two hours to help him with his homework. It usually takes the typical hyperactive child four times longer to do his homework than the average child.

Harris has a great desire to learn. Because he works much harder at home to keep up with the other children, we try to recognize his efforts and praise him.

I found he could learn if I provided the proper setting at home, gave him opportunity, understanding, and patience, and prevented disruptions from the outside world.

## Improving Coordination

Although some hyperactive children are well-coordinated, many aren't. It often shows up in clumsiness; they may be classic cases of "two left feet" or "all thumbs". They often have problems walking, running, hopping, jumping, kicking, throwing, and balancing.

The poorly coordinated child usually has more difficulty doing little things with his hands and fingers. He has difficulty tying his shoes and buttoning his shirt. He has a poor pencil grasp when writing or has trouble folding paper exactly in half. These children sometimes benefit from special exercises.

If your child is poorly coordinated, encourage him to strengthen the weak areas by playing games that help develop muscle coordination. Toys like Legos,® Micronauts,® or Tinker Toys,® with many small pieces to manipulate, are good.

Electronic games (hand-held or video) improve eye-hand coordination. They sharpen reflexes, enhance memory skills, and relieve tension.

Drawing or writing letters is helpful. If the child writes letters to friends or relatives and gets one in return, he will be utterly thrilled.

Pencils, paper, and crayons should always be available, as well as other materials for creativity and self-expression. He can use paint, scissors, paste, modeling clay, fabric scraps, etc. Since children create emotionally, intellectually, and artistically, their art work frequently illustrates their innermost feelings.

## Oversupply of Energy

A child's overactivity reveals his oversupply of energy. He has to be constantly fidgeting, jiggling, rocking, banging, running, jumping, climbing, crawling — constantly on the move. He never walks when he can run and never sits when he can be up. He leaves a trail of disorder and seems to never tire out.

In addition, he has a passion for touching things, whether it be objects or other children. Twelve year-old Carrie can't walk into a room without touching everything in sight. Her fingerprints are left along the walls and on every piece of furniture. Each knick-knack has to be picked up and examined.

Such a child may be hyperkinetic, but his activity is so disorganized. He expends huge amounts of energy to accomplish nothing! After a brief rest, his battery is recharged and he is ready to go again. Come bedtime, he is never quite ready to give up at a reasonable time.

Harris, for example: Friday is the only night he gets to stay up late. He sometimes watches a late-night TV show. After much coaxing, he still tries to stay up as late as his body will allow. His eyelids become heavy from sleepiness. He falls asleep in the chair. One morning when I asked why he fell asleep in the chair, he answered, "I can't keep my eyes open. They keep shutting on me."

## Impulsiveness

Much of the trouble the hyperactive child makes can be traced to impulsiveness. He reacts too quickly. He needs to delay his responses. He needs to be taught the consequences of his actions. His impulsiveness makes him unable to restrain himself, but he needs to be taught to stop and think before he acts or talks.

By acting before he thinks he gets into trouble — lying, stealing, cheating or running into the street without looking. He leaps before he looks, regardless of the outcome. He can destroy toys, clothing and other objects at an unbelievable rate. He can make a room come apart better than a cyclone. If his explosive temper does not get the best of him, his impulsive nature will.

Harris would get angry and tear at his shirt. The buttons would fly in every direction. Or he would throw objects — books, musical tapes, teddy bears, Legos, anything.

## No Predicting

The child is unpredictable. It's hard to know what to expect from one minute to the next. His moods are negative. Nothing seems to please him. Once he gets into his nasty mood, it is impossible to get him out of it. We have to wait it out. Even a "Good morning" can lead to an argument about what kind of a morning it is.

When we were planning to have dinner at the home of a friend, Kate Stewart, Harris announced, "I am *not* going!"

"Yes, you are," I said calmly.

"No, I'm not!" he spat out.

Knowing his unpredictable behavior and how he loses his ability to reason, I ignored the comment. Thirty minutes later, he asked, "Mom, what time are we leaving for Mrs. Stewart's?"

## Accident-Prone

We all have to expect a few bumps and bruises on our children, but the hyperactive child usually gets more than the average child. He is so accident-prone. He does not show fear during his perpetual motion, because he does not anticipate the dangerous outcome. Hence a hyperactive child requires closer supervision than other children.

His impulsiveness, lack of attentiveness, emotional upsets, and violent temper are key factors in his accidents.

## No Patience

Harris has a low frustration tolerance. He will destroy a toy or other object if he cannot make it work right away. When he couldn't get a bicycle part fixed, he would start screaming and kicking his bicycle. When he couldn't find a particular Lego® piece, he would throw all the pieces in the air in a fit of anger.

The hyperactive child may punch a friend over some minor thing. He will invariably pitch a wild temper tantrum when he can't get his way. He even gets so keyed up at happy events, such as parties, he spoils the fun for everyone.

Impatient should be Harris's middle name. It is a terrible trait of the hyperactive child. When Harris asks for something, he thinks I should immediately have it ready for him. He wants it right now, even though it's a spur-of-the-moment request.

Despite his impatience with others, he demands extreme patience from us. He can be a regular slowpoke, moving at a snail's pace. It is as if he mistakes the word "hurry" for "take all the time you want." He is so slow, he almost misses the school bus every morning. Just as the bus rounds the corner, Harris hustles out the door, still buttoning his shirt, with his shoes half-tied, lugging his backpack behind and parroting, "Mom! Did I forget anything?"

### Mile-a-Minute Talker

This child is such a chatterbox! It is difficult for anyone else to get a word in edgewise. He talks endlessly at top speed about anything and everything. He also has an irritating habit of monopolizing conversations.

This can create a problem because there are many people, like myself, who enjoy and value solitude. There is no way for the hyperactive child to be "turned off." He seems unable to talk in a soft voice, shouting all the time.

When Harris watches a TV show with Steven, he fires off questions like a machine gun. Steven can't listen to the show. It's the same with the rest of the family. Steven refuses to let Harris watch TV with him, unless Harris promises not to utter a word until commercial time. During commercials, Harris chatters away, but when the show starts, he clams up.

The hyperactive child usually laughs or talks in a loud voice, but not all do. The loud ones have poor muscular control of speech modulation, rhythm, and frequency,[4] which can involuntarily produce a high-pitched, tense voice.

### Poor Loser

No one likes to lose, but few people take a loss as hard as a hyperactive child. When he loses, he feels he has failed. He needs to realize that it is not a disgrace to lose, that it is not important to win every time, but it is important to enjoy playing. When a child wins all the time, he is not playing with children of equal ability. He has no real competition.

## Comrades

Every child needs friends, but it is difficult for a hyperactive child to have a friend for long. He loses friends because of his hostile behavior, destructiveness, selfishness, win-at-all-costs attitude, quick temper, and immaturity. Even though he might realize the reasons why he loses friends, he may not be able to do much about it.

He often fights with the other children. The aggression relieves his hostility. Other children will grow tired of his constant hitting, poking, fighting, "smart-mouth" and "show-off" behavior. They will grow impatient when he is not able to finish a game, or when he constantly moves and bangs about. He is unable to get along with other children, so he develops a "chip-on-the-shoulder" attitude. In turn, this only leads to more fighting and harsh words.

This is true of eight year-old Kirk. He fought and quarreled constantly with other children. He developed a "foul mouth." The other children disliked him intensely. He was always tapping his feet or tapping his hands on his desk or tripping children in the hall. He couldn't sit still. He was up and down constantly from his seat, either sharpening his pencil, going to the bathroom, getting a drink of water, or teasing other children.

Kirk was uncontrollable at school. Spanking had little effect. His teacher became his victim. When he was corrected, Kirk grew angry and punched the teacher in the stomach. As a result he was suspended from school.

## Broken Promises

The hyperactive child causes others much displeasure. Each unpleasant episode ends with a solemn promise never to do it again. But he soon does the same thing again, and will continue to do so. He may understand that his behavior is not normal, or he may not realize what he is doing. Again, he could just forget. He has a problem with his recent memory. There are so many stimuli reaching his brain simultaneously that they cancel each other out. Sometimes the most important response needed at the moment gets cancelled out.[5]

The hyperactive child often looks down on himself as being "dumb," "stupid," "a jerk," "friendless," "a blabbermouth," "different" or "unlovable." Although he feels guilty about his bad behavior and all the trouble it causes, he is still unable to control his feelings and emotions.

For example, when Harris didn't know the answer to a simple problem, he always shot back "I'm a jerk!" or "I'm so stupid! Everybody knows the answer to that!"

He often said, "I'm a blabbermouth and that's why no one likes me." He constantly belittled himself over trivial things. Now that he is a changed person on his successful diet, he remarked only recently, "Mom, I know why I have so many friends now. I'm not a blabbermouth anymore."

These are some of the problems that plague the hyperactive child. It is easy to see that the child is severely handicapped by his symptoms and the negative response they inspire. His problems abound. But even the most challenged child can have some self-control, if he is given enough love, understanding, and intelligent care. We can influence the child's innately positive characteristics with specific techniques that will bring results.

We can look ahead to a brighter future for the child and ourselves.

# 19. Tackling Bad Habits

Harris's long, slim face was half hidden under his Pac-Man hat. His lips were quivering when he walked into the house with, "Mother, something awful happened today at the swimming pool. Roger broke his leg on the diving board and cut his head open. Blood was everywhere. They rushed him off in an ambulance."

My insides sank. After all, Roger was my best friend's son. I went to the phone to call her.

A mischievous grin spread across his face as he said, "Just kiddin'!"

Teasing again! I should have known better by now. Besides, his lips always quiver when he's teasing.

Bad habits. Those irritating things the hyperactive child seems to be great at — teasing, lying, stealing, cheating, starting fires, breaking toys, throwing things, avoiding chores, poor table manners, manipulating people, and countless others. These often drive us frantic.

Sometimes we simmer and stew and try to conceal our wicked feelings rather than make a big issue out of the irritations. Yet with constant exposure to them, our negative emotions continue to build up, like a ticking time bomb waiting to explode. We often think, "Oh, well, they'll go away."

What can be done? There is no magic wand trick to solve our problem. A bad habit must be coaxed out slowly, like going down stairs ... one step at a time.

It is also hard to attack the child's bad habits without attacking the child. Problems surface.

The following guidelines will help. They are not a prescription, but examples of ways of encouraging improvement, as well as ways that we ourselves can improve in certain areas to make the child's habit training easier. While the guidelines do not touch on every problem, they will provide ideas.

### Making the Switch

Although some of the physical reasons for your child's hyperactivity have been cared for, he may have learned some bad habits along the way. Often, when removing a bad habit, a parent should be prepared to accept a substitute. Consequently, when bad habits are broken or improved, they must be exchanged for more acceptable ones. It is best to work on only one problem at a time. Some little irritations can turn into major issues. Others can be handled easily, such as Harris's habit of breaking into the front of a line of people.

In our small town, the Fourth of July is the most celebrated event of the year. People come from miles around to join in the festivities. All kinds of games, fun booths, races, and other types of frolic take place for four days. Near the end of the celebration, the highlight is a "Destruction Derby."

One year, Harris and I found the waiting line for the Derby at least two blocks long. I refused to wait. Harris begged to attend because he was to meet his friends inside. I let him stay, knowing he would have to wait in the lengthy line.

When the Derby ended, I was there waiting for him.

"Harris," I sighed, "I sure felt sorry for you having to wait in that long line. How long did you have to wait?"

"Oh, I didn't have to wait hardly any time at all," he disclosed. "See, Mom, this is what I do: I go near the front of the line and stand by some people. The people in front think I'm with the people behind, the people behind think I'm with the people in front. No one ever says or thinks anything about it."

When I explained how unfair this is and why he shouldn't do it, he understood and promised not to repeat it. He had thought there was nothing wrong with the stunt. He confessed he had done it many times in the past.

## Home Front

A child will do best if he knows precisely what is expected of him. He should be a regular family member, taking on chores and responsibilities, as well as privileges. Each child should carry his load of the work as a part of the family.

Helping with chores can be an important factor in his psychological development. A child taught to do his best at home chores is learning to be a successful adult. Knowing he is needed and useful is gratifying and as important as feeling loved.

A parent should make a list of the chores the child can do, such as setting the table, walking or feeding the dog, making his bed, cleaning his room, taking the garbage out, doing yard work, etc.

It is important to remember that the hyperactive child will take more time to do the chores and may not do them as well as we would like. But we need to bite our tongues and stifle criticism. A child needs recognition and praise for effort.

When Harris first washed the dishes, he did a fairly good job of them, but not as good as I had hoped! He was slow. Likewise, with pulling weeds, raking leaves, vacuuming the car, and cleaning the bathroom. Nevertheless, he was trying to do a good job. Our lavish praise made him eager to do better.

Harris used to think that boys weren't supposed to help around the house. Once, when I asked him to perform a house chore, he declared, "You're the houseperson around here!" With help, his attitude has changed.

## Allowance

A hyperactive child's allowance should not be withheld as punishment or used as a bribe or reward — such as for performing a chore —or he may never receive one. (The exception is to withhold when financial payment is indicated to repair or replace damaged items for deliberate destructiveness.)

For example, suppose Casey vacuums. If his efforts are paid with money, then he will associate vacuuming with receiving money. So, if he is to dust, he will expect money for that too. When we produce the child's allowance on his satisfactory performance of chores, it gives him the feeling that he should be paid for every helpful thing he does instead of feeling that he should contribute to family life.

This also undermines the key purpose of an allowance: to teach a child how to manage and spend money and give him some independence. He won't learn to budget unless he can count on a regular sum. Therefore, he needs to be given a specific sum of money at regular intervals. Besides, how would we feel if our payday came around and our boss didn't pay us? A child's allowance is his payday.

It is not "our" money. Once we hand it over, it is *his*. We should not pry into how it is spent (unless it is for something harmful). The experience of spending extravagantly can be just as beneficial as spending wisely. We should not insist that he save his money. The decision to save should be his, not ours.

## Punching a Time Clock

The child needs to assume the responsibility of getting ready on time. When he is late, he must face the consequences. He needs to learn to act for himself when he is required to be at a certain place at a certain time. Drastic action is sometimes necessary.

It is also unfair to other family members when he is always late. It would be best to leave him home, but that is not always possible. He needs to know the negative result of being late and the positive for being on time.

Harris wakes up with ample time to eat, get ready for school, look for library books, put his belongings in a backpack, and catch the school bus. Instead, he waits until the last minute to get ready and misses the bus.

When this happens he rushes into the house with face flushed and hair mussed, still carrying the backpack he didn't have time to put on.

"Mom, I missed the bus! You have to take me to school!"

Since we live within a mile from school, I answer, "Today you will have to walk or ride your bike. I won't take you. You had plenty of time to get ready. You shouldn't have waited until the last minute."

The following morning, he makes more of an effort to get ready on time.

## Role Reversal

Often, the hyperactive child wants to control the entire family. He may get his way through violent temper tantrums, psychosomatic complaints or other bad behavior. If the parents usually submit, the other siblings complain that he gets away with murder.

Since his demands are always met at home, he becomes upset and unhappy when the same thing doesn't happen elsewhere. Parents should avoid this trap.

Six year-old Phillip often lies on the floor screaming and kicking when he can't have his way. His parents usually give in, but if they don't he suddenly develops a tummy ache or headache. Out of pity, they give in to him. When Phillip's parents recognized the control he had over them, they began to handle him differently. They stood firm, unwilling to submit to him. Not only has Phillip's conduct improved at home, he is also behaving better at school.

## Coping with Misdeeds

Constant lying requires us to ask ourselves if the child is being criticized and punished too much and is lying to avoid more of the same.

When we know for certain that the child has done a specific wrong, we should not ask him if he did it. He will impulsively deny the accusation. It is best to confront him with our knowledge so it can be discussed.

Take Wesley, for example. His dad becomes irate if he leaves his belongings in the living room. When Wesley leaves his books there, his dad gruffly asks, "Wesley! Did you leave your books in the living room again?"

"Daddy, I didn't put them there," the seven year-old stammers. "Someone else must have."

Because Wesley has been constantly criticized and punished for trivial things by his high-strung dad, he thinks his only way out is to lie or blame others. Finally, Wesley's dad changed his tactics. Now he is less critical and has stopped punishing Wesley for trivial things. He rewords his remarks. Instead of saying, "Wesley, pick up your books and put them where they belong," he will explain why Wesley should not leave his books in the living room. Result: Wesley feels no need to lie impulsively and he gradually starts accepting blame for his misdeeds.

## On the Road to Crime

Some hyperactive children help themselves to things that don't belong to them. This habit can lead to trouble. Each time the child steals and gets away with it, the bad habit is reinforced. This will cause serious trouble throughout life if he doesn't learn the rules of the game early. He has to understand he is responsible for his own actions and will have to suffer the consequences. Sometimes it helps to talk with the child. Explain to him *why* he should not steal someone else's property.

We have been on both sides of this fence. When Harris was eight, he and a young friend ventured into the drug store. With much coaxing from his friend, Harris stole a yoyo. He already had two at home. He was caught red-handed.

When the phone rang, I was shocked to hear:

"Mrs. Mitchell, this is Jim at the drug store. Harris and a friend were just here. Harris stole a yoyo. I reprimanded him and sent him home. I just wanted you to know. Perhaps you should talk with him. I didn't call the police. It's not that big of a deal. Besides, I felt the other boy was more to blame. He convinced Harris to steal it. The whole incident has Harris pretty shook up."

Harris came in crying hysterically. "What are you going to do to me?"

After explaining why he shouldn't steal and extolling the virtues of honesty, I marched him back to apologize. He then had to pay for the yoyo with his own money and put it in the handicapped children's box.

This incident was a blessing in disguise. It left an impact on Harris. He was terrified at having been caught and didn't want to go through that again.

On the other side of the fence, Harris was leaving for school with his bright new "nerf" football. It was still wrapped in plastic.

I suddenly remembered his name was not on it. I shouted, "Let me take off the plastic and write your name on it!"

"No, Mom," he replied. "I'll miss the bus. I'll take the plastic off at school and write my name on it."

He forgot. A friend stole the football. Harris was heartbroken. He knew first-hand what it felt like to have something stolen when he had to watch others play with it.

## Sporty Events

Sports and games play a significant role in developing children's value systems. Certain sports allow the child to release an enormous amount of energy and some require little discipline. But the hyperactive child should never be pushed into a sport when he is unwilling. He will be embarrassed if he fails in front of others. As a result, he will dislike himself even more.

Harris goes for sports with constant action, such as soccer, football, or basketball. He refused to play baseball, and we don't push the issue. He sits on the sideline and watches.

Parents who feel their child will never shine athletically shouldn't push him into failure. Let *him* make the choice.

## Music Therapy

The hyperactive child must have an outlet for his enormous energy. The exploration of music can provide a means of self-expression, either with musical instruments or voice. Music is a good tension-reliever because the child can literally work off pent-up feelings through rhythmic action.

It takes discipline to practice a musical instrument, so it may be hard on him to follow through. Nonetheless, he will do better at anything when it is shared by his family.

## TV is Harmful

A child who spends hours watching TV during his formative years will leave childhood with fewer verbal and logic skills than one who spends those hours playing, sharing, drawing, reading, listening, talking, exploring, and learning.

The child in front of the TV screen is not achieving or exercising his body and mind. What's more, he may be picking up bad habits.

Research shows that a lot of TV watching affects the child's school performance, learning ability, play activities, attitude, and behavior.

In a study by Sharon Gadberry of Adelphi University, the six to eleven year-old children who were heavy TV viewers put in much less effort at schoolwork than light viewers. If a child simply must watch TV, time should be limited.

Bad habits can be added to the lengthy list of reasons why hyperactive children are harder to raise, but they can be raised successfully. There are techniques to make the task easier.

# 20. Grapevine of Techniques

Several months before Christmas, our mail order catalogs already have become dogeared, torn, and marked up. Then comes a long list of desired toys, prices, and notes on which catalog carries the cheapest price tags.

This particular year, Harris and Steven had their hopes built on an expensive BMX race car set. It was far out of our price range, so the boys worked at odd jobs to help buy the toy.

When the exciting event drew near, we pooled our money and ordered the set from a local store.

We left the store toting the expensive, long-awaited toy, with both boys sharing the burden of carrying it. Eyes twinkled. Faces gleamed with enthusiasm. Hands trembled from excitement.

At home the box was quickly torn open as we all perched on the floor.

"Hurry, Daddy. Help us! We need you to put it together!"

Beau plopped down and joined our group.

"Where are the instructions?" he queried. "I have to have something to go by. I can't put it together right without them."

Eyes darted all around, but the instructions for the complex set had been accidentally left out of the box. Beau tried to put the race car set together without instructions. Progress was slow.

It was Christmas Eve and the stores had closed early. Beau called our friend, Marvin, who had put an identical set together for his son. For fifteen minutes, Marvin explained in detail how to assemble the set.

Under Marvin's direction, the pieces fell into place. When the contraption was assembled, we all felt a keen sense of accomplishment.

This experience is similar to raising a hyperactive child. No packet of instructions comes with him. (Believe me, I looked — there were none!) Harris relayed his "plan" to me.

He told me, "I'm not having any kids — they're too much trouble! If I do, though, I'll get rid of them when they reach about five or six." Later, as he repeated our conversation to a friend, he added, "But my mom says I won't want to get rid of them no matter what — I'll love them too much by then."

If there had been instructions with the child, they probably would have read: "Give lots of kindness, understanding, patience, and guidance. Correct him without crushing, help him without hanging on and give lots of love. Match with an equal amount of prayer." These are the tools for building a happy and successful child.

There are techniques to make raising the hyperactive child an easier task.

Our plans for the child parallel our plans for the race car set. We want the child to last long and run smooth, with the least amount of trouble. We want him to have a more positive effect on people so they will admire him and our well-done job. We want them to compliment him, enjoy him and want to be around him, even to want to take the child home for a visit.

## Methods Abound

The typical hyperactive child is not "sick," so parents can do a great deal for him. While some children need more extensive help than others, most parents can spot specific problems and learn to deal with them. This chapter includes many techniques to help parents handle their atypical offspring.

First, we have to learn to accept that which we cannot change and make the best of the situation. That's just the way it is! We must realize that each child is born with certain personality traits that he will carry with him throughout life. He probably will always have a high activity level. He probably will retain a certain amount of talkativeness, impulsiveness, impatience, and irritability. These are traits he must accept and then work on. Diet control will make this easier. We have to face reality. This is the way the child is and probably the way he always will be.

After we realize that the child has certain characteristics which cannot be changed, then we can help him accept himself. We need to accentuate the positive. I think everyone responds to the approach that he has problems, but everyone else has problems too. We must make the point that he is not alone.

When I informed Harris that Susy, who lives on the next block, is on the same diet, his eyes sparkled with surprise. A wide grin spread across his face. He was thrilled! He hadn't realized that other children have the same problems. He thought he was the only child on earth to be on the diet.

## Booster Shot

It is a good idea to explain to your child everything you know and have learned about his condition. You will relieve the child's anxieties by explaining the various problems and symptoms of the syndrome.

Let him know you realize it is difficult for him, and that you are aware of the many problems he faces each day. He needs to be reassured of his parents' love. He needs to know that you love him just as much, in spite of his problems.

Willie is an example. He is a hyperactive eight year-old with a multitude of problems. He brought nothing but heartache to his parents. Willie didn't think his parents loved him as much as they loved his sister, Rose. She never caused them grief.

Willie's parents carefully explained in a way he could easily understand that each person is different. Everyone has his or her own personal set of problems. Some are just not as obvious as others.

Then Willie's mother asked him, "Would you still love me as much as you love Daddy, even though I had more problems?"

"Of course!" he blurted.

Relief swept over him. Due to his fresh understanding, the problems appeared to dwindle.

Explain to the other children in the family what you know about the syndrome, too, and enlist their help. It will be hard for them, but they can be helpful and understanding. Besides, they need to know why there is a constant uproar in the household. It is important that they learn to make special effort to get along with the hyperactive sibling.

Sherry is an example. At fourteen she goes out of her way to cope with her nine year-old hyperactive brother, Tim. When he gets mad and calls her names, she turns a deaf ear. She says she knows his bad mood will pass and that basically, he is sweet, softhearted, and bright. She concentrates on his positive side and tries to ignore the negative.

## Accept Him

Acceptance of a child is essential to his self-esteem. Acceptance indicates we do not feel the need to make him over. We need to like, enjoy and respect him, and to value his many good qualities. Growing into an acceptable, responsible adult is hard enough when a child feels loved and wanted. The hardship is magnified for the hyperactive child.

It is easy for parents to accept a bright, cheerful, obedient achiever. It is much more difficult to accept a child who seems to constantly do wrong and seems hopelessly unreasonable in every way.

The child has to find acceptance with us before he will be able to find it with anyone else. Simply accepting the child does not mean we just ignore his bad behavior. It means we take him the way he is and we do the best with what we have.

We need to accentuate the child's positive qualities. Encourage and reward the skills and strengths he has, rather than focusing only on his negative traits and weaknesses. Sure, his pluses and minuses may be different from those of the child next door. They may not fit in with our own goals for him, but *he needs to find acceptance the way he is*!

The sweetest music to his ears is hearing his parent say, "I like you just the way you are." But some children, such as Skooter, wait for these words to no avail.

Marla, an unwed mother, reserved all her love and attention for only one of her two young children. The other child, five year-old hyperactive Skooter was totally neglected.

Marla expected Skooter to be like his sister, Kristi, an "ideal" child. At seven, Kristi required little attention. She was bright, kind, and well-behaved. She was easy to accept.

Skooter was the opposite. Marla was unprepared for her predicament. She found she was unable to accept him the way he was. She wanted to make him over but couldn't. Her feelings of hopelessness were turned on Skooter — short temper, screaming fits, and repeated spankings. Her behavior only made his worse.

## Mistaken Identity

On the other hand, some parents spend more time and attention on their hyperactive child than on the others. It is especially difficult for a non-hyperactive child not to feel left out and perhaps loved less when his parents pay more attention and perform more time-consuming tasks for their hyperactive child. The non-hyperactive child might also feel that the hyperactive child gets away with too much. Although some rivalry, jealousy and fighting is expected in every family, the non-hyperactive child often feels his parents love the hyperactive child more.

Billy is an example. At age eight, he thought his parents showed more love, worry, concern, and attention for his hyperactive seven year-old brother, Lee. Billy felt his parents treated Lee like a king, trying to fulfill his every whim and wish.

Billy thought he was required to do most of the home chores, while Lee lived an easy life. Billy became jealous and took his insecure feelings out on Lee. He picked fights with him, constantly tattled on him, hid his books, answered his phone calls and said Lee wasn't home when he was, and so on.

The key to understanding is communication. Parents need to explain to their non-hyperactive child why it is not possible for Lee to do the same chores Billy does. Lee is unable to perform the same chores. He is not as capable, although he seems perfectly able in every way. It should be stressed to children that every person should be judged according to what he is able to do. It is good to explain that parents expect more from a child without problems than they do from the hyperactive one.

All children need to feel secure in their parents' love. They need to be made to feel worthwhile themselves. Then they will naturally be more considerate, understanding, and sympathetic with the hyperactive child in the family.

## Good Self-Esteem is Necessary

The hyperactive child is especially vulnerable to low self-esteem, because of a vicious cycle of reasons. He is accident-prone. His behavior continually upsets others. In turn, he becomes depressed. He soon begins to belittle himself, regardless of his accomplishments.

Truth is, the extent of a child's happiness correlates with his degree of self-esteem, or the opinion he has of himself. Any child with a low opinion of himself is a handicapped child. The more he fails, the more his depressed self-image will hold him back.

Most parents are more concerned with their child's poor self-image than they are about his unruly behavior. This is as it should be. A child's self-love is essential to a rewarding life. A child is just not meant to continually say, "I'm no good," "No one loves me" or "Everybody hates me." When his self-esteem is built up, he will be able to tackle the world successfully.

He needs to believe he can succeed in the goals he sets for himself. Believing is the first step toward achieving. He needs to respect himself to be able to respect and love others. With confidence and assurance, he will be more charming to other people. They will then enjoy his company.

Often we parents nourish the bodies of our children and fail to nourish their self-esteem. Some parental attitudes lead to frustrating, self-destructive devaluations of a child's self-esteem. We should not apply constant, harsh discipline to every little thing the child does.

Explain to the child that no one is perfect. He will make mistakes just as everyone does. He should be honest with himself and improve when he can. But he should *never* believe he is a failure, unworthy of love and respect. If a child feels good about himself, he can take charge of his life. His "*I can*" might be more important than his IQ.

Once when Harris made a mistake, I reassuringly said, "Nobody's perfect!"

"Yup!" was his reply. "But everybody's more perfecter than me."

There's an interesting saying that goes like this: "If you had a bar of gold and continually called it lead, it would in no way change the quality of the gold. However, when a child is repeatedly belittled or talked about in a way that is less than he is, he begins to believe it."

We need to build up the child and not tear him down. One way we can do this is by telling him, "*You're somebody special!*" And mean it! Because he is.

A child who lacks friends will think poorly of himself. He will be deficient in self-love. The more his self-esteem is built up, however, the more friends he will be able to make and keep.

Look at Johnny, a hyperactive twelve year-old. He lost his parents in a car accident at the tender age of eight. He was shifted from one foster home to another. He developed a poor self-image, believing no one loved him because he couldn't find a real home and family. Children shunned him because of his problems.

Then a young couple adopted Johnny and gave him a warm, loving home. They were aware of his problems, but this didn't hinder the adoption. Johnny felt someone finally cared for him. Of all the other children, they chose him! He began to think better of himself and gained confidence. When he began his new school, he made friends easily.

## Rules to Follow

Experts agree that a clear set of rules and guidelines in the home is of great benefit to a child. One who grows up in a home where behavior limits are consistent is more likely to develop high self-esteem than one from a more permissive environment. The unregulated will often become unsure and worried about whether he is doing the right thing or not.

The hyperactive child needs to have a precise picture of what is expected of him in the home and outside world. He needs to know what to do and when to do it. He will then know when he is meeting expectations or when he is not. He should not have too many choices. They make him feel more insecure.

A rule is a guideline for anything we expect the child to do or not to do: the type of behavior he is expected to show and what is forbidden; any chore he is to perform or responsibility to fulfill. A good rule is one that is reasonable and can be easily understood and followed by the child. It should be enforced. Too many rules are just as bad as too few. It is important that the child always abide by the rules we set for him, as well as the rules of all mankind. He will suffer all his life if he doesn't learn to follow the basic rules of society.

## Independence is An Asset

The hyperactive child needs to learn he is responsible for his own actions. Then as he grows and matures, he should have more freedom to make his own choices. This will teach him responsibility so he can be more independent. He needs to learn independence so he will not be too dependent upon his parents. This is an asset that will help him triumph over his handicap.

Since he acts before he stops and thinks, he will do things he will regret. He will test rules because of his adventurous nature. He will be subject to physical danger because of his impulsiveness.

Despite his impulsive nature, we should not constantly defend the child but let him take responsibility for the way he acts. Help him acknowledge what a difference the new diet makes, but do not allow him to blame his misbehavior on what he eats. He needs to learn to control his own body.

## Love = Discipline

The hyperactive child often gets more discipline than the average child (although his siblings may not think so), but often it is less effective. He can't concentrate long enough to hear what he has done wrong or how to correct his behavior. Much is due to his uncontrollable urge to move around, which leads to a greater chance of accidents. He may also have a reduced response to pain. His fearless foolishness can be a problem.

Parents who run a disciplined home usually have a sense of direction. Discipline provides structure in a child's life. We should discipline constructively and consistently. Set few rules, spell them out clearly and enforce them. We should be reasonable, understanding, fair, and flexible. It is important for us to bear in mind that either we teach the child discipline or the world will teach him in a way destructive to his happiness.

Security and stability come most easily to those who have been loved within their homes. Our parental authority should not be totalitarian. It does, however, need to be patient, kind, gentle, open-minded, and understanding. Our discipline should be based on love and not on personal caprice.

Every child needs to know when his behavior is unacceptable, but there are various ways we can go about doing it. We should speak frankly, expressing our feelings and dislikes for the child's antisocial behavior. Be reasonable and consistent. But we should *never* compare his bad behavior with the good behavior of another child.

This is what happens to seven year-old Amy. Her mother constantly compares her to her problem-free sister, Janice. The mother often complains, "Why can't you be like Janice? She's nice and everybody likes her!" This kind of comment only heightens Amy's already sad condition.

Simple commands delivered in a firm voice are more effective than empty threats. Threats only cause more stress for the child.

Six year-old Michael's high-strung father, David, fits the saying, "his bark is worse than his bite." When he becomes upset with Michael, he screams frightening threats, like "If you don't stop dropping your food on the floor I'm going to call your friends over and whip you in front of them" or "I'll tell your friend, Leah, that you wet the bed."

Although David is a softie under his rough exterior and would never do what he threatens, Michael takes his threats seriously. It puts unnecessary stress on his body, and only aggravates his problem.

We should try to display a positive mental attitude. If we feel confident, the child will feel likewise. Do not give the child an indecisive answer. State exactly what should be done and see that he does it — even though you might not feel that decisive.

A confident person avoids nagging, screaming and threatening.

Rules and punishment for breaking them should be stated clearly. *Then stick to it! Don't budge!* This may seem like a hard-nosed approach, but it is the best way.

Sally, the mother of ten year-old twins, recounts: "Thursday, I tell them I want every weed pulled in the garden anytime before dark. If it's done on time, they can go to a movie Friday night with their friends. If it's not done, or is done wrong, they will stay home and work on the weeds. They know from testing me that I'll keep my word."

## Tuning In

Communication is a two-way street. It is sometimes more important to listen to the child than it is to talk to him. We need to offer a sympathetic ear. By active listening, we are offering him our acceptance of his feelings. This means a great deal to a child. For this reason, we need to keep the "phone" line open with the "receiver" ready for listening.

This realization struck me when Harris said, "Mom, did it ever occur to you that I just like to talk with you — not about anything in particular — but you're always too busy?"

It is good to show physical gestures of affection. The child needs contact with us — a hug, a kiss, holding hands, sitting on our lap, or just touching in some way. These are all ways of communication.

We need to eliminate criticism in the child's life. Criticism is a form of child abuse — mental abuse. Instead, we should praise him more so we can help build his self-esteem. We need to remember that listening is better than preaching, encouraging is better than scolding, and suggesting is better than demanding.

A troublesome child often has too many pressures. He is unable to accept any criticism (he probably gets too much), is negative, uncooperative, and frequently bursts into tears or wild temper tantrums. He thinks no one likes him. He is irritable most of the time. He thinks of himself as a failure. He says he wishes he had never been born, and has nothing good to say about anything or anybody.

What's more, his peers, teachers and even his parents often act negatively toward him. He needs a close relationship with his parents. He wants love and acceptance from them, but often finds they don't listen to his problems.

## Have Flexible Goals

We need to help the child reach the behavior goals set for him. These goals must be flexible and realistic, not too high.

Monte, a hyperactive teenager, said, "My older brother, Rod, always makes straight A's, but I can't. I am just not capable of it. Even if I studied constantly, I still couldn't. My dad expects too much from me. He thinks I should be like Rod. He fumes, fusses, and restricts me if I make anything less than A's. He won't settle for B's. He gripes if I make F's and he gripes if I make B's. So why even try?"

We will always have to make allowances for the temperamental differences between this child and another one. We must realize that just because one of our other children made a certain accomplishment by a certain age, does not necessarily mean that the hyperactive child will be able to do so. Everything appears to take more time for these children.

## Praiseworthy

We should always praise the child for his accomplishments. He desperately needs it. His disorder is a real burden on him and he needs constant encouragement. A hyperactive child can be trying and exasperating, even though he is loved. But the hyperactive child will respond to warmth, gentleness, sincerity, understanding, concern, and love.

Words of praise to a child are almost as important as love, kindness, concern and affection. A good passage to heed from Haim Ginott, is, "If you want children to improve, let them overhear the nice things you say about them to others."

A warm smile, a word of praise, a hug, a kiss, a pat on the back, a hand on a child's head or a special reward lets a child know his efforts to do the right thing pay off. They show him that we are happy with his efforts.

Each of us likes praise, appreciation, and recognition for doing the right thing. Some parents are generous with their compliments and affections and show their love lavishly. This is as it should be.

Often, however, we parents fail to notice when the child does well and we take his good behavior for granted. We make no special effort to comment when he keeps out of trouble, yet we are quick to notice when he does badly. A child will learn more from praise than criticism.

## No Way to Shield

There is no way we can shield the child from the many cruel and thoughtless things other people will say about him. Although he does many things to displease and disappoint us, we should not make it a habit of believing the worst about him from others. Just because he *usually* is guilty does not mean he always is. Therefore, we should not automatically side with other people, especially before letting him defend himself.

Mary is an example. She is the mother of Craig, a hyperactive eleven year-old. She left him outside the grocery store while she went in to shop. When she returned, she found the police talking with a woman whose car had been backed into another vehicle.

A child, it seems, saw the keys in the ignition, got into the car, started it up, put it in reverse, and rammed it into the other vehicle. The only problem concerning Mary was that Craig was the accused. A teenager said he witnessed the accident and specifically identified him.

Mary said her first thought was, "That's just like that rotten brat!" Her temper flared. Craig cried hysterically and repeatedly said he didn't do it. Mary said that for a few seconds she felt like tearing him limb from limb, but she finally regained her composure.

"I put myself in his shoes," she confessed. "Suppose *I* told *him* the truth about an incident and yet *he* believed a total stranger whom he had never seen before instead of believing *me*, whom he loved. I decided to treat him as I would want him to treat me. When I finally told him I believed him, I never saw a kid so flushed with relief."

## Label Stickers

It deeply hurts the hyperactive child to be branded by labels, such as "hyperactive," "behavior problem child," "troublemaker," "slow learner," "learning disabled" or "socially maladjusted." These labels often become part of his self-concept. Thus he tends to live down to these bleak diagnoses. Although *everyone* has problems, many are disguised and are not so obvious as this child's.

Parents should never label their child as "hyperactive." Once he is labeled, it seems like everything that goes wrong is blamed on him. It's sadly unfair.

Ruth learned this first-hand. Barry, her hyperactive seven year-old was accused by their neighbor, Mrs. Gregg, of pushing all her potted plants off the porch and smashing them with a crowbar while she was gone for the day. Barry denied the misdeed. Still, Mrs. Gregg insisted to Ruth that he had. "After all," she stormed, "you said he's hyperactive!"

Even other children may begin labeling the child as "hyper," "crazy," "wild," "stupid" or "dumb." This will only lower his already poor self-image even more. He will begin to see himself as others see him and will belittle himself. This is what happened to Harris.

Each morning when the "special" bus came by to pick up a mentally retarded child on the same block where Harris caught his bus, it passed by him, and the other children waiting at the bus stop. Some children shouted that *Harris* should be on the bus for the mentally retarded because that's what he was! They stuck the label "retarded" on him. The sad part is that he actually began to wonder if he was.

## Love Him in Spite of . . .

Hyperactivity does become a negative factor in raising a child, but the child has to feel he is wanted and loved in spite of the problems he may have. Surprisingly enough, he might be convinced that not only do his parents not love him, but that he is *unlovable.* He has feelings of rejection and is burdened with shame because he knows he does so many things to distress and disappoint us.

Furthermore, he might feel that other family members only see him as a nuisance and seem relieved when he is not around. He may also feel that his brother or sister dislikes or even hates him. As a result, he will have no respect for himself.

He may want desperately to make his family love him, be happy, pleased and close to him, yet he has little control over his bad behavior.

There are many ways we can demonstrate our love for the child: by taking an interest in his well-being, by establishing rules and by seeing they are carried out; by showing concern for him; or by looking out for his welfare, such as by knowing where he is or when he will return home. These are all ways of showing we are interested and care about him. It warms his heart with joy.

For example, Steven and Harris. During the summer months, they often go to the park and spend the day, either swimming or playing around the park. We have them phone home every few hours so we will know they are all right.

Anytime either one leaves home, he is expected to tell us exactly where he is going and when he will return. If he is a little late, we start calling or go and look for him.

No parent should allow his or her entire life to revolve around the problems of one child. This is more than the parent or the child can endure. Besides, a parent might have other children who need attention. It is best for a parent not to show favor to a particular child, even though one child might require more time than another one.

We must not treat the hyperactive child like he is handicapped and give in to his every little whim and wish. It will only make it that much harder for him. It won't be helping us either.

The child is an important part of our lives, but still only a part. We must not allow him to become our whole life. It isn't fair to the child to expect *him* to provide *us* with a sense of self-worth.

As his hyperactivity appears to diminish, don't be tempted to allow him more leeway. That may prove to be a big mistake. It's tough living on a day-to-day basis with a hyperactive child, but that's the only way it can be done.

## Love Conquers All

Underneath, the hyperactive child is actually kind, warm, goodhearted, sympathetic, compassionate, and lovable — much more so than he may get credit for. This is why it is so important for us to constantly reassure him of our love.

Reassurance of love is like the first Christmas card Steven gave Harris.

It read: "For a wonderful brother" on the front. Inside it said, "I love you."

Harris's blue eyes lit up like another ornament on the tree. He was ecstatic! His brother loved him! Harris set the beautifully inscribed card on his dresser, where it sat for many months. When I asked why he didn't put it away, he answered, "'Cause it reminds me that my brother loves me."

Just as surely as a child needs the proper food to grow, develop and function properly, he needs mega-doses of "psychological vitamins," like "You're such a good boy," "I love you so much" or "I'm proud of you."

The hyperactive child needs our supportive help. He is frightened of the outside world and he desperately needs our full support. He needs to feel victory from some of his accomplishments. He also needs to hear encouraging words from us. He hears enough discouraging words from the outside world.

Most of all, he needs to feel enthusiastic and cheerful about living, because he is wanted, loved, and accepted. This would make anyone's life more pleasant. And as long as we love and care for the child, there is hope.

## Postscript

The recipe for a healthy, happy, calm child is varied, but here are some key principles to remember:

1. Avoid sugar.
2. Be prepared! Always have something wholesome and satisfying ready to eat.
3. Feed your child often — about every two hours.
4. Never give a child any form of sugar (refined or natural) on an empty stomach.
5. For sweet snacks or desserts use only fruits. They should never be eaten without some form of good quality protein.
6. Nutrition is best guaranteed when a variety of foods are consumed.
7. Be a label reader.
8. Calcium and magnesium calm many hyperactive children.
9. Vitamin C fights colds and infections.
10. Accept your child for what he is. Try not to compare him to others.
11. Be consistent, but firm, in discipline.
12. Be generous with love and compliments.
13. Pray!

# PART V
# Morsel Tips and Recipes

# 21. Yuk to Yum Morsels

Following are some ideas for morsels to get you started shifting over to a diet to help conquer hyperactivity. Listed first (Quick Treats) are some of the items your child can eat safely now, unless you are aware of an allergy or sensitivity to the foods in them. Remember, for the best progress avoid sugars. Even fruits, which include a form of sugar, should not be eaten excessively.

Listed second (Tasty Combos) are some of the items your child can eat if his sensitivity has been checked and he has no adverse reaction to these foods. The list includes milk products and salicylate-containing foods, which may cause problems for some children. Refer to Appendix A for more information.

## Quick Treats

1. Hard-cooked, shelled egg.
2. Tuna, egg, or chicken salad in celery sticks.
3. Peanut butter or other nut or seed butter in celery sticks.
4. Cooked fish or chicken.
5. Popcorn — use kelp or sea salt as a seasoning, or sprinkle with nutritional yeast.
6. Jello with unflavored gelatin, fruit chunks, and fruit juice.
7. Deviled egg made with homemade mayonnaise or mayonnaise without additives and sugar.
8. Peanut butter as a dip for celery, cauliflower, or raw vegetable.
9. Nuts and seeds such as peanuts (really a legume), walnuts, pecans, almonds, filberts, cashews, brazil, soybean nuts, pumpkin seeds, and sunflower seeds. These are also good all mixed together.
10. Raw vegetables with a dip.
11. Half herb tea with half fruit juice.
12. Peanut butter mixed with wheat germ on whole grain bread.
13. Tuna fish, chopped carrots and bean or alfalfa sprouts.
14. Hot whole grain cereal for any meal.
15. Dried fruits such as pears, banana chips (no sugar added), or pineapple.
16. Peanut butter on whole grain bread or crackers sprinkled with sunflower seeds.
17. Sandwich with peanut butter, nuts, and banana slices.

18. Two whole grain crackers spread with nut butter and mashed banana to make a sandwich.
19. Unsweetened granola and fruit.
20. Cashew butter between carrot slices.
21. Chopped liver on celery or lightly toasted whole grain bread.
22. Herb teas, hot or cold. Emphasize water!

## Tasty Combos

1. Cheese between two thin slices of apple.
2. Cheeses with whole grain crackers.
3. One tablespoon cottage cheese scrambled into two eggs.
4. Cheese sandwich topped with sunflower seeds.
5. Cucumber boats filled with egg, tuna, or chicken salad.
6. Skewers of cheese cubes, avocado, cherry tomato; fruit skewers made of apple chunks, orange wedges, banana slices, cherries, grapes.
7. Peanut butter and berries instead of peanut butter and jelly sandwiches.
8. Cored apple with cream cheese or peanut butter.
9. Add sesame seeds to salad (such as tuna or chicken salad) with cheese and sprouts on pocket bread.
10. Plain yogurt with mashed banana, pineapple, berries, or other fruit.
11. Cottage or ricotta cheese with grated pineapple.
12. Dried fruits — apples, apricots, peaches, raisins, or prunes.
13. Cottage cheese as a dip with raw vegetables — carrot, celery, cucumber, or zucchini.
14. Celery sticks with peanut butter or cream cheese and topped with raisins.
15. Cored apple stuffed with shredded cheese or homemade cheese spread.
16. Steamed cauliflower sprinkled with shredded cheese and chopped walnuts or sunflower seeds.
17. Chopped nuts or seeds in carrot and raisin salad.
18. Tuna with chunks of cheese and bean sprouts in whole wheat pita bread.
19. Cream cheese and walnuts on whole wheat raisin bread.
20. Cottage cheese with whole wheat crackers.
21. Applesauce stirred into plain yogurt.

# 22. Helpful Tips

Helpful tips are a lot like hugs — something we don't have to have, but they make the going a whole lot easier. These helpful tips include ways to retain the most nutrition from foods, some food storage and food preparation time-saving techniques, and ways to utilize ingredients that otherwise might be discarded. I think you will find these tips will help you win the never-ending kitchen marathon.

1. Add extra nutrition to baked items with nutritional yeast, wheat germ, lecithin granules, kelp, peanuts, chopped nuts, and seeds. Bran will add extra fiber.
2. Pears, instead of apples, for pies, sauce, cookies, muffins, etc.
3. Reduce honey in recipes and substitute part or all with fruit juice concentrates.
4. If honey granulates, reliquify by placing the uncovered container in a pan of hot water. Do not boil.
5. When baking with honey, warm it first in a pan of warm water. It will blend into the dough easier.
6. Light coating of liquid lecithin instead of grease on pans or cookie sheets will keep foods from sticking.
7. To leach calcium from soup bones, use something acidic like tomatoes, vinegar or lemon juice. After cooking and calcium is leached out, discard bones.
8. Unsweetened pineapple juice as the liquid instead of water when making applesauce. It will be sweet enough without adding sugar.
9. If you run out of buttermilk, add a tablespoon of lemon juice or vinegar to a cup of milk.
10. Add nutritional yeast to baked goods, casseroles, juices, shakes, smoothies, or sprinkle on foods such as popcorn or salads.
11. Nuts and seeds, shelled or unshelled, keep best in the freezer.
12. Refrigerate natural nut and seed butters to keep the oil from separating.
13. Keep all whole grains refrigerated.
14. Use carob powder ounce for ounce as chocolate.
15. Dilute fruit juices with water.
16. Date sugar as a natural sweetener.
17. Wheat germ or oatmeal in meatballs.
18. Soybean milk instead of cow's milk, if there is no sensitivity.

19. Soybean curd (tofu), grated, diced, cubed or sliced into hot dishes. Also may be blenderized to creamy consistency for use in cooking.
20. Wheat germ in cereals.
21. Add liver to chili, which hides the taste of almost anything.
22. Sprouts instead of lettuce on sandwiches.
23. Nuts or seeds in such salads as tuna, egg, chicken, or cole slaw.
24. Nuts, seeds or fruits in a school lunch.
25. Coconut in peanut or other nut butter.
26. Fruit in nut butters.
27. Yogurt instead of sour cream.
28. Save water left over from cooking vegetables for soups and stews.
29. Tofu in pancake mix.
30. Pancakes with soybean milk. Add nuts or seeds.
31. Grated carrots in meatloaf.
32. Nuts or fruits in homemade ice cream.
33. Soybean milk in ice cream instead of cow's milk.
34. When measuring honey, molasses, syrup, peanut butter, or other thick, sticky ingredient in a recipe, measure oil first. The contents will then slide out of the measuring cup without sticking.
35. Don't peel vegetables, scrub them. The greatest concentration of nutrients are usually in the peel and just under it.
36. Bake cakes, cookies, pies, muffins, etc., with fruits, vegetables (pineapple, bananas, pears, carrots, zucchini), oatmeal, or a nut or seed butter.
37. For every cup of flour required in a recipe, replace two tablespoons with a like amount of soy flour. Because wheat (a grain) and soy (a legume) contain complementary proteins, this combination will enhance the protein value of baked goods.
38. Grate rinds of whole citrus fruits, spread out on a tray, and freeze. (Wash well first, if not organically grown.) Transfer to airtight containers. They will keep for months. When ready to use, thaw them at room temperature for one hour — or add them frozen to cold drinks. They can be used for tea, or garnishes for all kinds of dishes, or added to baked items.
39. Citrus fruits will yield more juice if they are rolled beneath your hand on a counter top before squeezing.
40. Store raisins in the refrigerator for up to two years. They will retain flavor, color, and nutrition. Better yet, freeze them.
41. Freeze small cartons of yogurt. Put them in the lunch pail straight from the freezer. They will keep the rest of the child's lunch chilled and be thawed by lunchtime.

# 23. Quick and Easy Recipes

A specialist first suggested that we give a child two tablespoons of peanut butter when he arrives home from school. It works like this: Open the child's mouth, shove the peanut butter in, and close. Push him into a closet — wait thirty minutes. Out will come an altogether different child.

I gave it a try and sure enough it works! Of course, I don't go so far as to push Harris into a closet, but I do manage to get the peanut butter down. It perks him up and gets him into a pleasant mood after a stressful day at school.

Quick, easy, high-quality recipes are a great help. The following are just such recipes.

1. Frozen banana on a stick, coated with carob powder, wheat germ or peanut butter.
2. "Bananapear" — ¼ pear topped with 1 tablespoon peanut butter and topped with a banana slice.
3. Fruitsicles out of fruit juices, diluted with water. Eat as popsicles.
4. Fruit juice with chunks of fruit frozen in popsicle molds.
5. Mashed banana with coconut and chopped nuts.
6. Tahini with equal amounts of a nut butter and grated coconut, made spreadable with frozen pineapple juice.
7. Homemade pizza crust, baked and spread with shredded cheese, peanut butter, and sunflower seeds. Bake ten minutes until cheese melts; also good sprinkled with raisins. (Pizza freezes well.)
8. Orange yogurt popsicles: Mix together 1 pint plain yogurt, 1 6-ounce can undiluted frozen orange juice concentrate and 2 teaspoons vanilla. Freeze.
9. Chef salad roll-up: Spread a leaf of romaine lettuce with mustard or mayonnaise. Top with strips of cooked chicken, turkey, or beef. Add cheese, sprouts, or any raw or cooked vegetable. Roll up tightly and secure with toothpicks.
10. Slice 4 to 6 pieces of fruit into bite-sized chunks; mix and top with ½ cup plain yogurt, flavored with nutmeg or cinnamon.
11. Nutritious topping: Mix 1 to 2 teaspoons frozen orange juice concentrate with yogurt.
12. Banana peanut butter pops: Mix 1 cup milk, 1 banana cut into chunks, ½ cup peanut butter, 1 teaspoon vanilla. Blend and freeze in popsicle molds.

13. Peanut butter spread: Mix together 2 tablespoons peanut butter, 2 teaspoons honey, 1 teaspoon wheat germ, 1 teaspoon sunflower seeds, 1 teaspoon raisins, 1 teaspoon unsweetened granola.
14. For a topping or spread: Mix 1 cup softened cream cheese with 1 tablespoon honey, topped with raisins and chopped walnuts.
15. Spread small amount of peanut butter inside pitted dates. Insert a brazil nut in the center of each date, close, shake in a clean bag with carob powder.
16. Spread nut butter on bread. Add grated carrot and raisins; or add apple butter and coconut flakes; or wheat sprouts and chopped dried apricots.
17. Roll frozen banana halves in 1 tablespoon melted crunchy peanut butter and then in 1 tablespoon toasted wheat germ.
18. Banana spread: Add a little lemon juice to a mashed banana, add chopped raisins and chopped sunflower seeds.
19. Sandwich spread: Work to a creamy consistency 4 ounces cream cheese with a little orange juice, add 1 tablespoon grated orange rind, then work in finely chopped raisins and grated coconut.
20. Fill dates or figs with mixture of cream cheese, wheat germ, chopped nuts, and a touch of grated orange rind.
21. Waldorf salad: Combine 2 cups diced, unpeeled apples, ½ cup diced celery, and ⅓ cup chopped walnuts. Use plain yogurt with a touch of honey for dressing.
22. Avocado dip: Two mashed avocados with a little lemon juice, sea salt, a little mayonnaise or tofu, chopped onion, and garlic to taste.
23. Ground oat flour: Place 1¼ cups rolled oats in a blender or food processor. Cover and blend about one minute. Makes 1 cup ground oat flour.
24. Wheat germ, bran, lecithin granules, nutritional yeast and cinnamon (optional), pre-mixed for sprinkling on soups, salads, casseroles, vegetables, pancakes.
25. Mix an assortment of fresh vegetables and stir-fry. Start with about 2 tablespoons vegetable oil and heat in a wok or large skillet. (I use a cast-iron skillet.) Add cut-up vegetables, herbs, or spices and stir-fry over medium heat. Stir constantly until vegetables are desired tenderness. (The crisper, the better.) A small amount of water can be added if needed to prevent sticking. Variety of combinations is limitless!
26. Cook beans with relief from the side effects (gas): Soak raw beans in water for two to three hours. Throw out the water. Cover the

beans with boiling water. Cook for thirty minutes. Discard water. Cover with fresh water, cook until tender.
27. Prepare a trail/snack mix chock-full of nutrients. I make a big batch and freeze it for use as needed. This makes nice gifts. I use one-fourth or one-half cup each of the following items, but you can vary amounts, or add other items not listed. Raw nuts and seeds are best:

> Peanuts, pecans, cashews, almonds, filberts, brazil, pumpkin seeds, sunflower seeds; unsweetened flaked coconut, chopped dates, raisins, carob chips; any dried fruit such as banana chips, apples, peaches, apricots, pineapple, papaya; granola is another option.

28. This is a simple recipe we devour quickly. Banana and pineapple are the least problem-causing foods.

### Easy Carob Treats

¼ cup carob powder
1 cup peanut butter
1 medium-ripe, mashed banana
¼ cup sesame seeds or chopped nuts
¼ cup unsweetened shredded coconut (optional)

Combine ingredients and mix well. Form into a log, about 1½ inches in diameter. Wrap in waxed paper. Store in freezer until ready to eat. Slice off desired amount and return remainder to the freezer.

## Creative Salads

The best salads are created with a little imagination, wit, culinary ingenuity, and a sense of color and design. A salad need not be merely iceberg lettuce and tomatoes. Those taste good, but you should go further. Experiment with other greens for fresh taste appeal, excitement, variety, and health-giving nutrients.

Add all sorts of vegetables to make a *real* salad — just as you would add colors to make an attractive painting. The more you vary the colors, the more balance you will have in the nutrients.

Salads can be the most stimulating and luscious part of your meal. Take advantage of Nature's bounty and put the spotlight on your salads. They will contain a superabundance of vitamins and minerals, as well as fiber and enzymes. But don't make the mistake of peeling the vegetables and tossing away that nutritional gold. Scrub them clean and keep the peels intact. If you feel you must peel, then take off a very thin layer.

Mix up an array of vegetables (almost any vegetable edible when cooked is good raw in salads) and add anything from shredded or cubed cheddar, jack, or Swiss cheese, chopped or sliced hard-cooked eggs, tofu, nuts, seeds, legumes (particularly garbanzo and kidney beans), seasoned whole-grain croutons — whatever strikes your imagination. Sprouts will contribute a whole symphony of nutrients and flavors. You can use alfalfa, mung, lentil, rye, wheat, garbanzo, radish, sunflower, adzuki or fenugreek. Avocado or herbs are good, too.

Be inventive and you will create your own masterpieces to tantalize anyone. Your new concoctions will be wholesome, flavorful, eye-catching, and crunchy. Vary the salad makings from day to day. Change prevents boredom. If your child has a salicylate sensitivity, eliminate cucumbers, green peppers, tomatoes, cider and wine vinegar from your salads.

## Finishing Touch

Now for the salad dressing. Some people wouldn't dream of eating a salad without a dressing. You don't want to smother a cool, crisp salad with a thick goo. Dressing must be selected with the same care you would give to the choice of a scarf or a tie. The simpler the dressing, the better. Try making your own dressings, using oil and vinegar, yogurt, or mayonnaise as a base. Flavor with herbs, spices, fruit juices. Use the least amount of dressing that will satisfy your family's palates. Don't have the dressing slopping around in the bottom of the salad bowl. The salad dressing is the finishing touch that determines the final character of your creation.

## Creative Shakes and Fruit Smoothies

Secret weapons — protein drinks: Mix your own ingenious shakes and fruit smoothies. They are powerhouses of nutrients and healthy replacements for sugar-sweetened shakes. For most drinks you can use frozen banana chunks. They do double-duty as sweetener and thickener.

Peel ripe bananas, cut into chunks (about six per banana) and freeze. Mix different fruits or "powerpackers," two or more when possible, in each drink. You can throw in whatever you like. Possibilities are boundless.

**Basic directions:**
1. Depending on the recipe and how many it will serve, blend a base of ½ to 1 cup or more milk, soy milk, yogurt, buttermilk, nut/seed milk, fruit juice.
2. Add three to six frozen banana chunks, more if needed.
3. Add what you like from the following list. Blend all ingredients in a blender until thick and smooth. Adding more frozen banana chunks or another frozen fruit (such as strawberries, chopped peaches) will make it thicker.

## List of Add-ins

Fruit juices: Apple, apricot, cranberry, grape, orange, pear, pineapple.

Fruits (fresh or frozen): Apple, apricot, avocado, banana, cantaloupe, cherry, cranberry, dates, figs, grapes, kiwi, lemon, lime, nectarine, orange, papaya, peach, pear, pineapple, plum, prunes, raisins, strawberries or other berries.

Sweeteners: Barley malt, carob powder, unsweetened coconut, date sugar, honey, molasses, pure maple syrup, rice syrup.

Flavorings: Pure almond extract, pure lemon extract, pure vanilla extract, cinnamon, nutmeg, etc.

Power-Packers: Nutritional yeast, kelp powder, lecithin granules, protein powder, nuts/peanuts and their butters, sesame/sunflower seeds and their butters, sprouts (all kinds), tofu, wheat germ, raw egg, cottage or ricotta cheese.

**Samples:** 1 cup pineapple juice, about six frozen banana chunks, 2 tablespoons peanut butter.

1 cup milk, about six frozen banana chunks, 2 teaspoons carob powder, 1 tablespoon sesame or peanut butter, 1 tablespoon lecithin granules, ½ teaspoon vanilla.

½ cup soy milk, about four to five frozen banana chunks, ½ cup strawberries, a slice of pineapple, 1 tablespoon wheat germ.

1 cup apple juice, about six frozen banana chunks, 2 tablespoons chopped almonds, 1 tablespoon coconut, 1 tablespoon nutritional yeast.

Positive changes rarely are easy, but they do bring their own rewards.

The other day, as I was preparing dinner, Harris stood watching me cut up vegetables. Conversation evolved around his diet and his new lease on life because of it.

Harris, smiling so brightly and his blue lights filled with love, unexpectedly turned serious and said, "I don't know how you did it but I know *why*." His words hung quietly in the air for a moment. Then he squeezed me tightly. "Thanks, Moomhead."

My spirits lifted to the sky! Too choked up to speak, I let him know with my eyes and my smile how happy his words had made me. What more could I have asked for as a reward?

---

### Write Me About Your Child

I have taken a personal interest in helping children other than mine plagued with hyperactivity and/or a learning disability. After you have followed some of these ideas long enough to judge the results, I would enjoy hearing from you about your experiences (good and bad) with your own child. How was he or she before the program and after the program; what other steps you have taken toward helping your child?

I am interested in learning how you used some of the techniques described here, or perhaps developed some of your own. What was the most helpful in achieving your child's success? What foods set him or her off the most? Where were the greatest challenges?

This will be of considerable help to me — if I should decide to update this book or perhaps write another one concerning other experiences with a hyperactive and/or learning disabled child. By learning about your results and findings with your child, we could help others. Thank you.

Write me in care of this publisher.

# Appendices

## APPENDIX A: The Natural Way Program

### Foods to Avoid

Artificial Flavors, Colors, Preservatives, and other Additives
Sugar (except in fruits)
Milk and Milk Products (including goat's milk)
White Flour Products
Packaged Cereals
Junk Food
Candy and Soft Drinks
Chocolate and Caffeine

Dr. Lendon Smith notes, "If a food has a label, it is probably bad for you. Eat foods that rot, but eat them before they *do* rot."

### Food Additives

The number of foods and food additives that can cause allergic reactions are even more numerous than the symptoms they cause. Moreover, since they are never eaten alone, they can't be tested to see what effect they have on a particular child. This is why synthetic food flavors, colors and other additives should be totally eliminated from a child's diet. They can cause a number of childhood disorders — especially hyperactivity.

Chemical food additives are substances foreign to the hyperactive child's body. They are manufactured in a chemical laboratory. They are not part of man's natural food supply. Each synthetic food flavor or food color is a specific and chemically unique substance, each having different traits from the other. Any food additive can cause problems.

An additive-free diet excludes artificial flavors, colors and preservatives. Artificial or synthetic flavors and colors are in many, many foods that one would never suspect. This is why it is important to read labels.

Not all additives are bad — such as ascorbic acid. But to give you an idea of some of the chemical additives to be avoided, here is a review:

> Sodium nitrate, sodium nitrite; these are usually found in wieners, bacon, ham, or any of the cured, canned, or refrigerated luncheon meats.

> Sodium bisulfite, sulfur dioxide; these chemicals prevent the discoloration of dried fruit and inhibit the growth of bacteria.

BHT (butylated hydroxytoluene) and BHA (butylated hydroxyanisole); these chemicals prevent oils from going rancid. They are among the most frequently used additives.

MSG (monosodium glutamate)

Propyl gallate

Phosphoric acid

Phosphates; *Health Express* says, "Phosphates may well be a major causative factor of hyperactivity in the United States."[1]

## Sinister Salicylates

Intolerance to food additives and salicylates is not an immunological disturbance, so therefore it is not an allergy. It may resemble an allergy, but the two are not the same. There are no tests to determine an intolerance to a salicylate, just as there are none to test allergies to food additives. The only method available is to remove all the offending substances from the child's diet.

The substances called salicylates occur naturally in some foods (see list on page 179). Dr. Feingold found that some hyperactive children may be sensitive or intolerant to them. These substances are said to interfere with the chemical balance in the brain of some children with the result that the brain does not function normally. There is still controversy over this.

I am skeptical by nature and found all of this hard to believe. I experimented with some of the different salicylate-containing foods. As a result, I found several which plunged Harris into a negative mood.

Chili peppers, for instance. Beau loves them, so we always have them in the garden. After Harris had made some progress on the additive and salicylate-free diet, I made an avocado dip. Because Harris eats it, I usually leave out the chili peppers, but this time I added them.

Harris had been settled. His personality was loving and kind. When he ate the dip with peppers, he was thrown into an extremely negative mood, refusing to cooperate. At school the following day, he was no better. He was totally disruptive in his classroom and was hauled off to the principal's office. This made me more cautious in experimenting with other salicylate-containing foods.

## Avoid Salicylates

The foods containing salicylates should be totally eliminated from the child's diet in all forms for the best progress to be made. They can then be gradually introduced back into the diet, but only one food at a time (usually a favorite) for about a week. Watch to see what kind of a reaction he has, if any, from that particular food during that week. Each food must be tried separately. A child may be able to tolerate one food, but not another.

One major criticism of a non-salicylate food diet is that it excludes some of the common foods which are good sources of essential nutrients: for example, fruits, which are a good source of Vitamin C. Many of the fruits do have a high natural fructose sugar content, such as dates, raisins, figs, etc. But these should be eaten sparingly, if at all, whether or not there is a proven salicylate sensitivity.

Being on a non-salicylate food diet does not mean that a child has to stay off all these foods indefinitely. Some can be added back, or perhaps all of them, if no adverse reactions occur.

To my horror, I found that tomatoes belonged to this group. I never realized how many foods contain tomatoes until I excluded them from Harris's diet. They are in tomato sauce, ketchup, spaghetti sauce, pizza sauce, Bar-B-Q sauce, soups, stews, and many other everyday dishes.

When I introduced tomatoes back into Harris's diet, he appeared to have the classic signs of sensitivity. But upon excluding them and then reintroducing them, he showed no signs whatsoever. However, he eats them no more than once every four days.

## Natural Foods Containing Salicylates

| | |
|---|---|
| almonds | grapes and raisins |
| apples | wine and wine vinegar |
| apricots | green peppers and chilies |
| all berries | nectarines |
| cherries | oranges |
| cider and cider vinegar | peaches |
| cloves | plums and prunes |
| coffee | tangerines |
| cucumbers and pickles | tea |
| currants | tomatoes |
| oil of wintergreen | |

## Fruits Containing No Salicylates
These are the *only* fruits allowed

| | |
|---|---|
| bananas | grapefruit |
| pears | lemons |
| pineapple | lime |
| melons | |

## Drugs with Salicylates

| | |
|---|---|
| Aspirin | Medications with aspirin added |
| Aspirin compounds | Liniments |

White Tylenol (acetaminophen) tablets may be used as a good substitute for aspirin, since they contain no salicylates.

## Foods to Eat

| | |
|---|---|
| Whole Grains and Whole Grain Cereals | Such as barley, bran, bulgur, buckwheat, corn, millet, oats, rice, rye, triticale, wheat or wheat germ. |
| Good Quality Protein<br>Nuts and Seeds<br>Eggs | Fish, poultry, lean meat or liver. Legumes such as peas, peanuts, beans, soybeans, or lentils. Nut and seed butters; |
| Fresh Vegetables | Preferably raw, steamed or stir-fried. |
| Fresh Fruits | Eat the fruits rather than drink the juices. Not as concentrated and more satisfying. Should be eaten with a protein food. Avoid excessive amounts. |
| Fruit Juices (unsweetened) | Mix half juice and half mineral water or water. Drink with a protein food. Avoid excessive amounts. |
| Bottled Mineral Water<br>Herbal Teas<br>Water | These should be substituted for the soft drinks that may have been consumed before. |
| Carob | An excellent substitute for chocolate. |
| Sweeteners | Fruits or fruit juice concentrates are the preferred choices. If you *must* use a sweetener besides the two shown, use only the *bare minimum of one of the following*.<br><br>Blackstrap molasses, barbados molasses, sorghum, honey, pure maple syrup, barley malt, rice syrup. |

## APPENDIX B: The Vitamin Alphabet

### Fat-Soluble

The four fat-soluble vitamins, A, D, E and K, are measured in International Units (IUs). These fat-soluble vitamins, which are found in nature, are stored like fat in the body, mainly in the liver. Unlike the water-soluble vitamins, these vitamins can be toxic, potentially dangerous if taken in large amounts. The greater danger for most people, however, is inadequate intake.

The fat-soluble vitamins often need the presence of fats and minerals and, sometimes, one another to be absorbed properly from the digestive tract. These vitamins are more stable in heat than the water-soluble vitamins and are less likely to be lost in cooking and processing. Lack of adequate bile impairs absorption.

### Water-Soluble

These include the B-complex vitamins and Vitamin C, which tend not to accumulate in the body. Each is rapidly absorbed, circulates freely in the body and is then quickly excreted in the urine. Regular replenishment of these vitamins is necessary. The danger of toxicity is reduced as there is little risk of build-up in the tissues. The B-complex vitamins should always be taken as a group.

Synthetic vitamins are from chemicals made in a laboratory. Natural vitamins are made from foods themselves, like vegetables, grains, fruits or fish oils. Chemists say that all vitamins are the same, and that the body doesn't know the difference in a natural or a synthetic one.

Although they might be identical, molecule for molecule, *nature does not grow synthetic vitamins.* I recommend natural vitamins. In natural plants and other nutrient sources, vitamins do not appear singly but in combination with other co-factors (synergists) which help those vitamins to be assimilated by the body. On the other side of the coin, the synthetic vitamins appear in a single form only, without synergists.

Purchase only vitamin supplements without sugars, artificial flavorings, colorings, preservatives or other synthetic ingredients. *Read the labels!*

### Units of Measure

1 gram = 1,000 milligrams
1 milligram = 1,000 micrograms
International Units (IU)

## Vitamin Requirements
### U.S. Recommended Dietary Allowances (RDA)

| VITAMINS | RDA |
| --- | --- |
| **Fat-Soluble:** | |
| A | 5,000 I.U. |
| D | 400 I.U. |
| E | 30 I.U. |
| K | not established |
| **Water-Soluble:** | |
| $B_1$ Thiamine | 1.5 mg. |
| $B_2$ Riboflavin | 1.7 mg. |
| $B_3$ Niacin | 20 mg. |
| $B_5$ Pantothenic Acid | 10 mg. |
| $B_6$ Pyridoxine | 2 mg. |
| $B_9$ Folic Acid | 400 mcg. |
| $B_{12}$ Cobalamin | 6 mcg. |
| PABA (Para-amino Benzoic Acid) | not established |
| Choline | not established |
| Inositol | not established |
| Biotin | 300 mcg. |
| C (Ascorbic Acid) | 60 mg. |
| P (Citrus Bioflavonoids) | not established |

## Vitamin A

**RDA:** 5,000 I.U.

**Fat-Soluble:** Can be stored in the body and could be toxic.

**Bodily Functions:** Helps the body fight infection, especially of the respiratory tract. Necessary for proper growth of bones, tooth structure, nails, and healthy skin. Helps to maintain healthy condition of the outer layers of many tissues and organs. Helps prevent night blindness and poor eyesight. Essential for pregnancy and lactation.

**Deficiency Signs:** Increased susceptibility to infections, especially respiratory. Defective teeth, gums. Loss of appetite, vigor. Dry, rough skin. Night blindness, itching, and burning eyes. Fatigue, weakness, allergies, sinus trouble. Retarded growth.

**Natural Sources:** Beef liver, kidney, fish, eggs, milk, butter, cream and cheddar cheese, carrots, cantaloupe, papaya, apricots, peaches, sweet potatoes, squash, dandelion greens, lettuce, parsley, collards, swiss chard, fish liver oils.

**Helpful Information:** Stress or infection would suggest increasing the dosage. Vitamin E, $B_2$ and zinc make Vitamin A more effective on tissues. Bile salts, lecithin and fats are necessary for absorption of A. Mineral oil blocks absorption.

## Vitamin D

**RDA:** 400 I.U.

**Fat-Soluble:** Can be stored in the body and could be toxic.

**Bodily Functions:** Essential to prevent pyorrhea, tooth decay, rickets. Necessary for utilization of calcium and phosphorus for bone and tooth development. Needed by the parathyroid glands to control calcium level in blood. Very important in infancy and childhood.

**Deficiency Signs:** Lack of normal bone development in children. Softening of bones and teeth. Muscular weakness, lack of vigor. Fatigue, nervousness, arthritis. Burning sensation in mouth and throat. Retarded growth. May lead to rickets.

**Natural Sources:** Formed in body on exposure to sunlight. Milk, butter, eggs, fish liver oils, sprouted seeds, sunflower seeds, mushrooms.

**Helpful Information:** Increase dosage of Vitamin D, calcium and phosphorus after fracture of bone injury.

## Vitamin E

**RDA:** 30 I.U.

**Fat-Soluble:** Can be stored in the body and could be toxic.

**Bodily Functions:** Helps in formation of normal red blood cells, muscle and other tissue. Controls rate of fat breakdown in tissues. Helpful in blood cholesterol reduction. Protects fat-soluble vitamins and pituitary, adrenal and sex hormones. Prevents scar tissue formation, such as burns and sores. Protects against muscle degeneration. Dilates blood vessels and helps circulation. Protects lungs from air pollutants. Helps delay aging process. Necessary for healthy reproductive organs. Prevents calcium deposits in blood vessel walls. Protects against some forms of anemia. Can reduce varicose veins, hemorrhoids, pain of exercise cramps and rectal cramps. Calms restless legs. Assists in normalizing blood viscosity and maintains normal permeability of capillaries. Natural anticoagulant. Can be used instead of hormones after hysterectomy. Increases effectiveness of Vitamin A.

**Deficiency Signs:** May lead to increased fragility of red blood cells, problems related to reproductive, muscular or cardiovascular systems — strokes, heart disease, pulmonary embolism, sterility, or enlarged prostate gland. Retarded growth in children.

**Natural Sources:** Whole wheat, nuts, legumes, wheat germ oil, vegetable oils, eggs, butter, whole grain cereals, dark green vegetables, liver, raw or sprouted seeds.

**Helpful Information:** Should be spaced eight to ten hours apart from iron intake as each interferes with absorption of the other. Mixed *tocopherols* is the best choice; natural vitamin E, in a single capsule, including alpha beta, gamma, and delta tocopherols.

## Vitamin K

**RDA:** Not established.
**Fat-Soluble.**
**Bodily Functions:** Essential for production of prothrombin (aids blood clotting). Important to liver function. Can reduce prolonged menstrual flow and lessen cramps.
**Deficiency Signs:** Internal bleeding, increased incidence of hemorrhage. Delayed blood clotting.
**Natural Sources:** Soybean oil, cow's milk, egg yolk, kelp, liver, tomatoes, alfalfa, cauliflower, spinach, cabbage, kale, algae seaweeds, and other green plants. It is manufactured in the intestines by normal bacteria.
**Helpful Information:** Individuals who have decreased or no intestinal bacteria after antibiotics can suffer Vitamin K deficiency because the body depends on daily synthesis of this vitamin in the intestinal tract. Yogurt, kefir, or acidophilus can restore bacteria.

## Vitamin $B_1$
### Thiamine

**RDA:** 1.5 mg.
**Water-Soluble.**
**Bodily Functions:** Essential for normal functioning of nerve tissues, muscles, heart. Necessary for carbohydrate metabolism and normal functioning of digestive system. Aids body growth and repair. Stabilizes appetite. Essential in growth of learning capacity. Helps control emotions. Helps calm hyperactivity.
**Deficiency Signs:** Loss of appetite, mental instability, forgetfulness, feelings of persecution, confusion, irritability, weakness, lassitude, nervousness, insomnia, fatigue, vague aches and pains. Impairment of the cardiovascular system, numbness of hands and feet, mental depression, digestive disturbances, loss of weight, shortness of breath, and constipation. Beriberi. Can cause an increase in pain and noise sensitivity. May cause impaired growth in children.
**Natural Sources:** Brewer's yeast, brown rice, whole wheat, oatmeal, blackstrap molasses, fish, nuts, beans, organ meats, pork, fruits, eggs, milk, raisins, and avocados.
**Helpful Information:** Increased amounts may be needed to counteract the effects of stress or diuretics, if taken regularly.

## Vitamin $B_2$
### Riboflavin

**RDA:** 1.7 mg.
**Water-Soluble.**
**Bodily Functions:** Assists in metabolism of carbohydrates, fats, amino acids. Aids nervous system. Essential for building and maintenance of all body tissues. Improves growth. Essential for healthy skin, eyes and mouth. Controls eye's sensitivity to light. Improves antibody and red blood cell formation. Controls skin disorders, such as eczema. Promotes iron absorption.
**Deficiency Signs:** Inflammation of the mouth. Red, sore tongue, cracking of the corner of the lips, itching, and burning eyes. Fatigue, poor appetite and digestion, bloodshot eyes, dizziness, cataracts.
**Natural Sources:** Liver, kidney, milk, cheese, eggs, whole grains, nuts, blackstrap molasses, salmon, oysters, leafy green vegetables, and brewer's yeast.
**Helpful Information:** Any digestive disturbance or stress would require increased amounts.

## Vitamin $B_3$
### Niacin

**RDA:** 20 mg.
**Water-Soluble.**
**Bodily Functions:** Called the "fatigue-fighting" vitamin. Essential for good nervous system and circulation. Maintains normal functioning of the gastrointestinal tract. Prevents pellagra. Promotes growth. Necessary for metabolism of sugar (helpful during withdrawal phase). Maintains normal skin conditions. Decreases headaches. Improves concentration, appetite. Controls canker sores and halitosis. Can help schizophrenics.
**Deficiency Signs:** Pellagra, affecting skin, gastrointestinal tract, and central nervous system. Fatigue, mental depression, muscular weakness, irritability, loss of appetite, neuritis, loss of weight, insomnia, diarrhea, nervousness, mental disease, skin lesions, halitosis, chronic headaches, digestive disorders, and general weakness.
**Natural Sources:** Milk, butter, liver, lean meat, fish, brewer's yeast, wheat germ, brown rice, nuts, sunflower seeds, peanuts, legumes, green vegetables, potatoes, mushrooms, and whole wheat products.
**Helpful Information:** Niacinamide is more generally used than niacin as it is less likely to cause burning, flushing, and itching of the skin. But niacinamide does not lower the level of fats in the blood, as does niacin. The difference between the two, chemically, is that niacin contains an organic acid group and niacinamide contains an amino group.

## Vitamin B$_5$
## Pantothenic Acid

**RDA:** 10 mg.
**Water-Soluble.**
**Bodily Functions:** Helps build body cells, maintain normal skin and central nervous system. Necessary for normal digestive processes. Helps cope with stress. Contributes to metabolism of carbohydrates, fat, and protein. Helps adrenal glands produce cortisone and other hormones. Prevents premature aging. Helps allergies and some forms of arthritis. May ease sore and aching muscles.

**Deficiency Signs:** Increased susceptibility to infection, personality changes, mental depression, intestinal disorders, loss of appetite, weakness, eczema, constipation, muscle cramps, diarrhea, fatigue, duodenal ulcers, loss of hair, premature aging, restlessness, low blood pressure, asthma, dizzy spells, burning feet, kidney trouble, respiratory infections, allergies, hypoglycemia, and retarded growth.

**Natural Sources:** Pork, beef, liver, kidney, brewer's yeast, wheat germ, bran, whole grains, peas, beans, peanuts, egg yolk, broccoli, cauliflower, cabbage, green vegetables, and mushrooms.

**Helpful Information:** Pantothenic acid, with the other B vitamins, Vitamins A and C, should improve an allergy regardless of its cause.

## Vitamin B$_6$
## Pyridoxine

**RDA:** 2 mg.
**Water-Soluble.**
**Bodily Functions:** Essential to the nervous system. Aids in formation of red blood cells, food assimilation, and protein and fat metabolism. Maintains sodium-potassium balance for nerves and skin. Aids in antibody production. Necessary for healthy teeth and gums. May reduce discomforts of menstrual cycle. Safe diuretic. Prevents nausea during pregnancy. Allows liver to metabolize female hormones. May improve conditions for which cortisone drugs may be needed. Prevents various nervous disorders and is known to improve memory.

**Deficiency Signs:** Nervousness, irritability, depression, loss of memory, anemia, loss of muscular control, acne, insomnia, dizziness, arthritis, hair loss, weakness, skin eruptions, convulsions in babies, and learning disabilities.

**Natural Sources:** Liver, kidney, meat, fish, whole grains, wheat germ, brewer's yeast, corn, egg yolk, blackstrap molasses, bananas, cantaloupe, cabbage, milk, pecans, and green leafy vegetables.

**Helpful Information:** Raw foods contain more B$_6$ than cooked foods, as it can be destroyed by heat. Anxiety and the craving for sweets can be controlled with increased amounts of this vitamin. Women taking oral contraceptives need increased amounts of Vitamin B$_6$.

## Vitamin $B_9$
## Folic Acid

**RDA:** 400 mcg.
**Water-Soluble.**
**Bodily Functions:** Works with Vitamin $B_{12}$ in production of red blood cells. Maintains nervous system, intestinal tract, and white blood cells. Contributes to development of antibodies. Needed for normal growth. Helps healing process. Promotes healthy skin and hair. Aids in protein metabolism. Blood builder.
**Deficiency Signs:** Macrocytic anemia — lack of mature red blood cells; instead, they become larger than normal with less hemoglobin than normal. Fatigue, depression, insomnia, constipation, digestive disturbances, impaired circulation, graying hair, restless legs, reproductive disorders, growth problems, diarrhea, and birth deformities.
**Natural Sources:** Milk, liver, kidney, salmon, oysters, tuna fish, whole grains, nuts, legumes, dates, brewer's yeast, asparagus, lettuce, mushrooms, Irish potatoes, and green leafy vegetables.
**Helpful Information:** Only a small amount is needed. As much as 0.1 mg. is easily obtained from food. A prescription is needed for the 1 mg. size.

## Vitamin $B_{12}$
## Cobalamin

**RDA:** 6 mcg.
**Water-Soluble.**
**Bodily Functions:** Commonly known as the "red vitamin." Effective in small dosages, so expressed in micrograms. Necessary for production of red blood cells. Essential for normal functioning of all cells, particularly bone marrow, nervous system, and the gastrointestinal tract. Promotes appetite and helps metabolism. Promotes growth. Improves fatigue and weakness, and leaves a feeling of well-being. $B_{12}$ shots may be helpful in controlling allergies, stress or loss of appetite. Helps prevent certain forms of anemia.
**Deficiency Signs:** Pernicious anemia, nervousness, general weakness, loss of mental energy, fatigue, poor appetite, growth failure in children, sore tongue, apathy, and tingling of extremities.
**Natural Sources:** Virtually absent from all vegetable food sources. Only meat or animal products — and some brewer's yeast (check the label) — can supply Vitamin $B_{12}$. Liver, kidney, fish, meat, milk, milk products, and eggs.
**Helpful Information:** Oral contraceptives may reduce Vitamin $B_{12}$ levels in the body. The mineral, cobalt, is essential for the body to utilize Vitamin $B_{12}$.

## PABA
### (Para-amino benzoic Acid)

**RDA:** Not established.
**Water-Soluble.**
**Bodily Functions:** Helps in utilization of adrenal hormones and estrogen. Facilitates production of folic acid. Acts as part of co-enzyme system. Can keep hair from turning gray. Effective in burn pain control. Needed for healthy skin.
**Deficiency Signs:** Extreme fatigue, eczema, gray hair, headaches, constipation, anemia, depression, digestive disorders, reproductive disorders, and irritability.
**Natural Sources:** Brewer's yeast, wheat germ, whole grains, organ meats, eggs, yogurt, milk, and blackstrap molasses.

## Choline

**RDA:** Not established.
**Water-Soluble.**
**Bodily Functions:** Regulates liver function. Promotes normal fat metabolism. Minimizes excessive fat in liver. Assists in synthesis of certain hormones, such as epinephrine. Promotes manufacture of thyroid hormones, nervous system function, and helps prevent cirrhosis of liver. Reduces cholesterol and high blood pressure. Aids growth.
**Deficiency Signs:** Atherosclerosis, high blood pressure, heart trouble, impaired liver and kidney function, may result in cirrhosis of the liver, intolerance to fats, and poor growth.
**Natural Sources:** Lecithin, brewer's yeast, wheat germ, legumes, organ meats, fish, egg yolk, and green leafy vegetables.
**Helpful Information:** Choline, with inositol, is used in the internal manufacture of lecithin, which is believed to help remove damaging cholesterol from walls of arteries and dissolve it in bloodstream.

## Inositol

**RDA:** Not established.
**Water-Soluble.**
**Bodily Functions:** Protects against cardiovascular disease. Helps reduce blood cholesterol. Aids in metabolism of fat. Can prevent thinning of hair. Aids growth.
**Deficiency Signs:** High cholesterol, hair loss, eczema, dermatitis, poor appetite, and constipation.
**Natural Sources:** Brewer's yeast, meat, milk, nuts, citrus fruits, wheat germ, whole grains, lecithin, and legumes.
**Helpful Information:** Inositol, with choline, is used in the internal manufacture of lecithin, which is believed to help remove damaging cholesterol from walls of arteries and dissolve it in bloodstream.

## Biotin

**RDA:** 300 mcg.
**Water-Soluble.**
**Bodily Functions:** Necessary for intermediate metabolism of carbohydrates, fats, and proteins. Maintains sweat glands, bone, nerve tissue, blood cells, skin and hair tone.
**Deficiency Signs:** Skin disorders, dandruff, hair loss, eczema, mental depression, drowsiness, confusion, insomnia, extreme fatigue, anorexia, loss of appetite, low grade anemia, nausea, muscle pain, heat abnormalities, paralysis, lassitude and high cholesterol.
**Natural Sources:** Liver and other organ meats, brewer's yeast, whole grains, peanuts, beans, corn, soybeans, mushrooms, and eggs.
**Helpful Information:** Made by intestinal bacteria, so oral antibiotics, which tend to kill all bacteria may indiscriminately reduce supply.

## Vitamin C
### Ascorbic Acid

**RDA:** 60 mg.
**Water-Soluble.**
**Bodily Functions:** Important to formation of cells, tissue, nervous system, tooth, and bone. Helps repair of bone fractures. Aids formation and maintenance of capillary walls. Influences formation of hemoglobin, absorption of iron from intestinal tract, and deposition of iron in liver tissue. Necessary for proper functioning of collagen. Converts folic acid to folinic acid. Promotes healing. Aids in resistance to colds and infections. Protects body against viruses and bacterial toxins. Has diuretic and antihistamine action. Required by adrenal glands to produce hormones needed to fight stress. Maintains strength in blood vessels. Necessary for healthy teeth and gums. Sharpens mental abilities. Protects circulatory system against fatty deposits.
**Deficiency Signs:** Scurvy, inflamed gums that bleed easily, tooth decay. Anemia, loss of appetite, muscular weakness, joint pains, capillary weakness, excessive hair loss, listlessness, lack of endurance, skin hemorrhages, eye hemorrhages, fleeting pains in legs and joints, easy bruising, poor digestion, premature aging, tender lips, thyroid insufficiency, atherosclerosis, nosebleeds, and low infection resistance. In children — restlessness and irritability.
**Natural Sources:** Not abundant in grains or most cooked animal foods (except liver). Citrus fruits, apples, bananas, strawberries, melons, currants, rose hips, peppers, cabbages, parsley, mustard greens, watercress, tomatoes, potatoes, and other green vegetables. Easily destroyed by cooking.
**Helpful Information:** Vitamin C works best if taken with rutin and bioflavonoids, found in white pulp of citrus fruits. Stress or infections require increased amounts.

## Vitamin P
### Citrus Bioflavonoids

**RDA:** Not established
**Water-Soluble.**
**Bodily Functions:** Prevents Vitamin C from being destroyed by oxidation. Strengthens walls of capillaries and regulates their permeability. Helps maintain the blood vessel wall. Prevents hemorrhaging. Acts as anticoagulant, thus may prevent strokes. Builds resistance to colds and infections. Helpful in hypertension, coronary thrombosis, arteriosclerosis, respiratory infections, hemorrhoids, varicose veins, rheumatic fever, anemia, edema, bleeding gums, and damage caused by X-rays.
**Deficiency Signs:** Capillary fragility. Appearance of purplish or blue spots on the skin.
**Natural Sources:** Buckwheat, peels and pulp of citrus fruits, especially lemon and orange. Fresh fruits and vegetables. Powdered pectin.
**Helpful Information:** *Bio-* means active, rather than inert; *flavonoid* means the crystalline substance which provides yellow color in foods, such as orange or lemon.

# APPENDIX C: Minerals are Essential

Minerals are normally called trace elements because they exist in such small amounts in the body. Minerals, like vitamins, are essential to a hyperactive child's well-being. They are needed for over-all mental and physical functioning. If a child has a shortage of just one mineral, his entire body machinery can become upset.

Many people take minerals for granted and believe it is more important to supplement the diet with vitamins. Truth is, the body can tolerate a deficiency of vitamins longer than a deficiency of minerals.

Minerals are similar to vitamins in many ways, yet are different in that they are inorganic chemicals — elements that cannot be produced by the body. Their only source is external, from food or supplementation. Vitamins, on the other hand, are organic compounds found in foods and in some instances produced by the body. Some minerals are involved in the production of vitamins in the body.

To a degree, more so than with vitamins, mineral ratios directly influence the availability of the minerals themselves. For instance, too much copper will lower zinc levels; high zinc will lower copper, lead and cadmium levels.

While all children require the same essential nutrients and the need for them is constant, the need for the same nutrients between two children may vary. Some might require less of some minerals and some might absorb one nutrient well, but not another one.

As with vitamins, mineral shortages can be reflected by distinctive signs, such as anemia, rickets, goiter and many others. This happened to Harris. He had iron-deficiency anemia, caused by an iron-poor diet. (One of Harris's doctors informed me that hyperactive children who take amphetamine-type drugs are prone to anemia). I began giving him iron-rich foods as well as iron supplements. Within a few weeks, he began to feel better.

Iron supplements, as in the case of anemia, may need to be continued for several months. It is important to remember that a child can get too much of a good thing. Excessive iron can cause harmful iron deposits throughout the body. Other minerals that can be toxic in excess are copper, iodine, chromium, lead, selenium, manganese, and zinc.

Some of the minerals required in larger amounts that are not toxic are calcium, magnesium, phosphorus, and potassium. Again, some vitamins and minerals are known to work together. For example; calcium and Vitamin D, selenium and Vitamin E, and magnesium and Vitamin $B_6$.

There are nearly thirty essential minerals. They are found in all tissues and fluids in the body, especially the bones, teeth, and cartilage.

Minerals have many important functions, such as influencing muscular contraction, calming the nerves, permitting other nutrients to pass into the bloodstream, helping with the healing process, stimulating the hormonal secretion of glands, serving as detoxifying agents, making strong bones and teeth, and controlling body liquids.

In short, minerals are essential for our children's health and well-being. If we shortchange them on minerals, our children will pay.

## Mineral Requirements
### U.S. Recommended Dietary Allowances (RDA)

| Mineral | RDA |
| --- | --- |
| Calcium | 800 to 1,200 mg., depending on age (see table below) |
| Chromium | not established |
| Copper | 2 mg. |
| Iodine | 100 mcg. |
| Iron | 18 mg. |
| Magnesium | 400 mg. |
| Manganese | not established |
| Phosphorus | 800 to 1,000 mg. |
| Potassium | not established |
| Selenium | not established |
| Sodium | 2 to 4 grams |
| Zinc | 15 mg. |

### Calcium

| Age | RDA |
| --- | --- |
| 4 - 6 years | 800 mg. (A quart of milk has about 1,140 mg.) |
| 7 - 10 years | 800 mg. |
| 11 - 14 years | 1,200 mg. |
| 15 - 18 years | 1,200 mg. |
| 19 and over | 800 mg. |

**Bodily Functions:** Gives structure and strength to the bones and teeth. Necessary for blood clotting, muscle contraction and relaxation, nerve transmission. Serves as a catalyst in many biological functions and regulates the permeability of the cell membrane. Potassium and sodium for muscle tone are balanced by calcium. Activates several hormones necessary to metabolism. Needed to activate enzymes (digestive juices). Calcium acts as a nerve tranquilizer to overcome irritability and grouchiness; a calming sedative agent for insomniacs, helps regulate the heart rhythm, and is vital to the nerves. Many hyperactive children, found to be deficient in calcium, are calmed when given the mineral and seem to handle stress better.

**Deficiency Signs:** All bone-related diseases, such as osteoporosis or arthritis, nerve-muscle excitability, nervous disorders, facial spasms, convulsions, stunted growth, rickets, muscle cramps, twitches, "charley horses," sleeplessness, depression, irritability, excessive or lengthy menstruation, abnormal sensation of the lips, tongue, fingers, and feet. Poor quality and malformation of bones and teeth.

**Natural Sources:** The main sources are bone meal or dolomite. Also milk and milk products, meat, fish, eggs, wheat germ, kelp, nuts, sesame seeds, sunflower seeds, beans, kale, spinach, cabbage, turnip greens, and other green leafy vegetables.

**Helpful Information:** In order to function, calcium must be accompanied with magnesium, Vitamin D, phosphorus, Vitamin A and C. Stomach acid influences calcium absorption. Calcium is absorbed rather poorly. Thirty percent or less of what is ingested is actually used by the body. About ninety-nine percent of the body's calcium is found in the bones and teeth. The remaining one percent is in soft tissues.

## Sources of Calcium Supplements

Bone Meal: a rich source of calcium and phosphorus; contains no magnesium.

Dolomite: contains calcium and magnesium.

Oyster Shell Calcium: usually recommended by Dr. Smith.

Calcium Lactate: a milk sugar derivative, considered to be one of the easiest forms to assimilate. The late Adelle Davis recommended these tablets for insomnia. She called them her "lullaby pills."

Calcium Gluconate: a vegetarian source. It is good, but the amount of calcium in it is relatively low.

Calcium Carbonate: most common and most readily available of all calciums.

Calcium Ascorbate: Major ingredient is ascorbic acid — Vitamin C with some calcium added.

Calcium Pantothenate: Major ingredient is pantothenic acid with some calcium added.

## Chromium

**RDA:** not established.

**Bodily Functions:** Activates enzymes needed in glucose metabolism. Required for carbohydrate metabolism. May help diabetic conditions. Increases effectiveness of insulin. Stimulates synthesis of fatty acids. Helps heart disease. Prevents and lowers blood pressure. Reduces cholesterol. Helps fight mental change accompanying senility.

**Deficiency Signs:** Glucose intolerance, particularly in diabetics. Hypoglycemia. Possible heart disease. Impaired growth.

**Natural Sources:** Best source is brewer's yeast. Others are hard water, liver, whole grains, wheat germ, rye, cheese, bananas, oranges, potatoes, spinach, mushrooms, and green peppers.

**Helpful Information:** A compound of chromium is the basis for the "glucose tolerance factor," believed to be a complex of chromium and nicotinic acid. Chromium has been associated with impaired glucose tolerance. "Glucose tolerance" refers to the body's ability to metabolize properly glucose (blood sugar — the primary fuel for body and brain). Good glucose tolerance means that blood sugar levels are kept within proper limits — not too high, not too low.

Chromium alone is not as effective as Glucose Tolerance Factor, nor is it absorbed as well as GTF, which is absorbed far better than any other form of chromium, and can immediately go to work as a partner to insulin.

GTF supplementation has shown significant value in treating the two main disorders of glucose tolerance — diabetes (hyperglycemia) and low blood sugar (hypoglycemia).

## Copper

**RDA:** 2 mg.

**Bodily Functions:** Acts as a component of many vital enzyme systems. With iron, it is necessary for the formation of hemoglobin. Essential to maintain the myelin sheath around the nerves, which act as an insulator, like insulation around wires. Assists the body to oxidize Vitamin C. Involved in protein metabolism and in the healing process.

**Deficiency Signs:** General weakness, anemia, heart damage, loss of or graying hair, skin sores and impaired respiration. Copper deficiency is rare. Most people seem to have too much copper in their body rather than too little.

**Natural Sources:** Best source: pears. Also seafood, meat, eggs, whole grain cereals, legumes, nuts, raisins, apples, grapefruit, plums, oranges, carrots, potatoes, and green leafy vegetables.

**Helpful Information:** Copper works in concert with zinc. Some people get too much copper because copper tubing carries much of our water supply.

## Iodine

**RDA:** 100 mcg.

**Bodily Functions:** Goes into the making of thyroid gland hormones, which help determine the body's metabolic rate or use of energy. Aids in the general growth and development of the body.

**Deficiency Signs:** Thyroid gland enlargement (goiter), low functioning thyroid gland, fatigue, restlessness, increased irritability, tremors, slow mental reaction, heart palpitation, dry hair, brittle nails, and obesity.

**Natural Sources:** Iodized salt, kelp, seaweed, seafood, fish liver oils, eggs, onions, turnips, spinach, garlic, and pineapple.

## Iron

**RDA:** 18 mg.

**Bodily Functions:** Needed for hemoglobin, the vital red blood cell pigment that carries oxygen to and removes carbon dioxide from the body cells. A component of enzyme systems, aids energy utilization. Helps maintain the body's metabolism, helps resist disease, and allows adequate functioning of the nervous system.

**Deficiency Signs:** Anemia, fatigue, exhaustion, depression, weakness, dizziness, poor memory, shortness of breath, lack of appetite, pale skin, headaches, and low resistance to diseases.

**Natural Sources:** Desiccated liver, liver, fish, oysters, meat, egg yolk, blackstrap molasses, brewer's yeast, wheat germ, whole grains, beans, raisins, prunes, figs, dates, peaches, apricots, bananas, seeds, almonds, parsley, spinach, leafy vegetables, and use of iron cooking utensils.

**Helpful Information:** Vitamin C aids iron absorption, as does hydrochloric acid in the stomach. Should be spaced eight to ten hours apart from Vitamin E intake as each interferes with absorption of the other.

## Magnesium

**RDA:** 400 mg.

**Bodily Functions:** Essential for calcium metabolism. Activator of many enzyme systems, necessary for synthesis of certain amino acids. With calcium and phosphorus, essential to formation of bones and teeth, and for normal body metabolism. A "co-enzyme" in the building of protein; helps keep the heart, nerves and muscles in good working order and the heart regulated. Reduces blood cholesterol, helps prevent kidney-stone formation, and may lower blood pressure. Can fight fatigue and help one cope with stress. Because of its calming effect, it will especially help a hyperactive child.

**Deficiency Signs:** Excessive irritability of nerves and muscles, depression, alteration of moods, disorientation, confusion, excitability, apprehensiveness, nervous twitches, spasms, convulsions and seizures, tremors, irregular heartbeat, weakness, and easily fractured bones.

**Natural Sources:** Dolomite, brewer's yeast, sesame, sunflower and pumpkin seeds, nuts, wheat germ, legumes, whole grains, kelp, seafood, milk, eggs, alfalfa, celery, beet tops, endive, apples, lemons, apricots, figs, dates, grapefruit, and green vegetables.

**Helpful Information:** Calcium and magnesium share many functions and should be used together in a ratio of two parts calcium to one part magnesium. Pregnancy increases the need for magnesium, as does alcohol, cortisone, diuretics, or too much sugar. About seventy percent of the magnesium in the body is in the bones. The remainder is in the soft tissues and blood.

## Manganese

**RDA:** Not established.

**Bodily Functions:** Necessary for proper functioning of many enzymes, especially those that metabolize glucose. Aids in chlorine and fatty acid utilization. Necessary for normal pancreas function and development, and for normal functioning of the central nervous system. Needed for normal bone structure. With copper and iron, it acts as a catalyst in formation of hemoglobin. Prevents sterility.

**Deficiency Signs:** Stunted growth, loss of muscle strength, fatigue, weakness, tremors, poor coordination, sterility, possible diabetes, bone deficiencies, asthma, and loss of sex interest.

**Natural Sources:** Brewer's yeast, wheat germ, whole grains, buckwheat, nuts, seeds, legumes, kelp, raw egg yolk, blueberries, oranges, grapefruit, apricots, brussels sprouts, spinach, and other green leafy vegetables.

**Helpful Information:** Manganese should be increased if one has a high phosphorus intake.

## Phosphorus

**RDA:** 800 to 1,000 mg.

**Bodily Functions:** Combines with calcium to give strength to bones and teeth. Necessary for the utilization of calcium and Vitamin D, and regulates release of energy from the "burning" of proteins. A constituent of myelin nerve sheaths, it is important to kidney and nerve functioning and production of hormones. Phosphorus assists in the metabolism of carbohydrates, and helps to manufacture lecithin. An important element in good brain function. Acts as a "blood buffer" to maintain pH.

**Deficiency Signs:** Nervous disorders, mental sluggishness, weakness, general fatigue, appetite loss, weight loss, stunted growth, irregular breathing, poor bone and tooth structure.

**Natural Sources:** Bone meal, brewer's yeast, whole grains, milk products, eggs, seafood, meat, poultry, legumes, seeds, most vegetables, and dried fruits.

**Helpful Information:** Phosphorus requires presence of calcium and Vitamin D for proper utilization. Absorption of phosphorus is hindered by aluminum hydroxide, main ingredient in popular antacid compounds. About eighty percent of the body's phosphorus is found in the bones and teeth, and the remainder in soft tissue. According to Dr. Smith, "Phosphorus is high in the Western diet and may contribute to the calcium deficiency that relates to hyperactivity." Developing a severe phosphorus deficiency is difficult, since this mineral is found in so many foods. Too much phosphorus cancels out the absorption of calcium, an important mineral that already is difficult to absorb.

## Potassium

**RDA:** Not established.

**Bodily Functions:** Contributes to muscle contraction and nerve transmission, acting with sodium to regulate fluids. Stimulates the kidneys, and joins with phosphorus to send oxygen to the brain. Essential to proper functioning of the digestive tract. Helps convert glucose to glycogen and is necessary for healthy adrenals.

**Deficiency Signs:** Muscular weakness, paralysis, tiredness, heart rhythm disturbances, muscle twitching, nervous disorders, gas, indigestion, constipation, sodium overload, high blood pressure, and hypoglycemia.

**Natural Sources:** Kelp, brewer's yeast, milk, nuts, seeds, whole grains, potatoes, prunes, raisins, oranges, bananas, and green leafy vegetables.

**Helpful Information:** Unlike sodium, potassium is found largely inside the cells. Sodium, sugar, diuretics, or stress will push potassium out of the body.

## Selenium

**RDA:** Not established.

**Bodily Functions:** The function of this trace element in the body is that of a synergist, a helper to other nutrients. Assists in the utilization of Vitamin E, essential for healthy nerves, muscles and the reproductive system. Helpful in detoxifying the body from harmful poisons, and may protect the liver from certain degenerative conditions. Only trace quantities are needed.

**Deficiency Signs:** Dysfunction of the body, especially the liver.

**Natural Sources:** Brewer's yeast, wheat germ, wheat bran, oats, brown rice, seafood, meat, liver, eggs, milk, broccoli, cabbage, onions, tomatoes, garlic, and mushrooms.

**Helpful Information:** Selenium with Vitamin E stimulates the immune system. A deficiency of selenium increases the body's need for Vitamin E. Dr. Smith remarks, "Areas of the country with low selenium levels in the soil have a higher-than-average rate of cancer and hypertension."

## Sodium

Diets are usually sufficient in this mineral.

**Bodily Functions:** Sodium is an essential component of many body fluids such as blood, tears, and perspiration. With potassium, it regulates the body fluids.

**Deficiency Signs:** Apathy, muscle cramps, mental dullness, weakness, breathing difficulties, and nausea. It can cause heatstroke in hot weather. There is usually too much sodium in the body, rather than too little.

**Natural Sources:** Table salt, kelp, celery, romaine lettuce, green leafy vegetables, eggs, and watermelon.

Helpful Information: An excess will push the potassium out of the body. Dr. Smith also explains, "Those who eat some dairy products and animal protein should *not* salt their food, as the diet provides more than enough sodium. Vegetarians may need some sodium."

## Zinc

**RDA:** 15 mg.

**Bodily Functions:** Essential to insulin and hormone reproduction. Helps in the normal function of tissue and metabolism of protein and carbohydrate. Necessary for activation of Vitamin A, for absorption and performance of vitamins, especially B-complex. Essential in the synthesis of nucleic acids. Necessary to more than twenty-five enzymes involved in digestion and metabolism. It helps the intestinal wall absorb food and is necessary for normal prostate function. Required for good sexual development, and promotes the healing of wounds and burns. A component of the eyes, it also helps form skin, hair and nails. Essential to the growth process, and a factor in regulating the appetite. It may stop body or foot odor, help control acne, and reduce tendency toward "stretch marks." It benefits hypertension induced by cadmium, a dangerous heavy metal.

**Deficiency Signs:** White spots on the fingernails, growth failure, hair problems, skin diseases, psoriasis, fatigue, decreased alertness, memory failure, impaired wound healing, loss of taste and smell, anemia, bone deformities, dysfunction of the reproductive organs, sterility, possible diabetes, and susceptibility to infection.

**Natural Sources:** Liver, meat, oysters and other seafood, milk, eggs, legumes, brewer's yeast, wheat germ, wheat bran, whole grains, sunflower seeds, pumpkin seeds, nuts, onions, and green leafy vegetables.

**Helpful Information:** Vitamin A must be present in order for zinc to be absorbed. Low zinc levels also worsen the effects of a Vitamin A deficiency. Zinc deficiency can be induced by high levels of copper, an antagonist. Extra zinc may be needed if calcium intake is high.

## APPENDIX D: Summary of Contributing Factors

The late Dr. Paavo Airola, America's foremost nutritionist and leading authority on holistic medicine, wrote: "On the basis of my extensive research of presently available scientific studies studies and clinical observations, here are the basic contributing factors of hyperactivity and learning disorders in children, in order of their importance:

1. Processed foods, drinks, or condiments that contain artificial colorings and flavorings, even so-called U.S. certified colors.
2. Other man-made chemicals, additives and preservatives — especially monosodium glutamate (MSG, also known as Accent'), sodium benzoate, butylated hydroxyanisole (BHA), and butylated hydroxytoluene (BHT); likewise, toxic chemicals present in polluted air, water, and food, especially lead, mercury, cadmium and carbon monoxide.
3. Refined white sugar and refined white flour and everything made with them. Excessive sugar in the child's diet contributes to the development of hypoglycemia (low blood sugar), which is one of the common contributing causes of hyperkinesis.
4. Caffeine-containing beverages, such as colas, tea, and coffee. Chocolate also contains caffeine.
5. Allergies. The most common allergens are: cow's milk and cheese, wheat (even whole wheat), eggs, chocolate, and citrus fruits and juices.
6. Hypoglycemia. Whether it is related to allergies, excessive sugar in the diet, or other causes, hypoglycemia is one of the common contributing causes of hyperkinesis.
7. Nutritional deficiencies. Many hyperkinetic children suffer from severe nutritional deficiencies, although they have plenty to eat. The average American supermarket-boughtdiet of overprocessed, canned, and frozen foods is so lacking in vital nutritive elements, especially vitamins, minerals, and trace elements, that it may lead to chronic nutritional deficiencies. Result: overfed but undernourished children.
8. Such environmental factors as loud noises or noise inaudible to the human ear (infrasounds), and artificial light, such as fluorescent room lighting. Studies show that changing the lighting to a type of light spectrum more like that of the sun improved the hyperactive behavior immediately.
9. Drugs. Many commonly used prescription and nonprescription drugs can trigger hyperkinesis in children.
10. Lack of authoritative discipline and clear, defined rules of family life and expected behavior. Children, even at a very

early age, must know exactly what is expected of them and what they can and can't do. Some system of reward for good behavior and punishment for misbehavior is a must. Undisciplined and left on their own, children feel neglected, disoriented, confused, and tend to react with irrational behavior.
11. Deprivation of love and affection. Sometimes, hyperkinetic symptoms, especially destructiveness, rebelliousness, and bad temper, are expressions of deep-seated feelings of insecurity and of being unloved or unwanted."

(The above excerpt is quoted with publishers' permission from Dr. Paavo Airola's book, *Everywoman's Book,* published by Health Plus Publishers, P.O. Box 22001, Phoenix, Arizona, 85028. 1981 edition, price $12.95.)

## APPENDIX E: Glossary

**Additive:** Substance, natural or synthetic, purposely added to foods to prevent spoilage, improve taste, appearance, and texture, or to enhance nutritional quality.

**Allergen:** Any substance that causes an allergic state or condition.

**Allergy:** Hypersensitivity to a specific substance (such as food, pollen, dust, etc.) or condition (as heat or cold), which in similar quantity does not bother others.

**Amino Acids:** "Building blocks" of which proteins are constructed. All proteins are composed of a combination of twenty-two amino acids. Fourteen of these — called the *non-essential* amino acids —can be synthesized in the body. The remaining eight —called the *essential* amino acids — must be provided in food if adequate nutrition is to be maintained. Animal proteins, such as meat, fish, poultry, dairy products, and eggs, contain reasonable amounts of all the essential amino acids plus a good supply of the non-essential ones. Therefore, they are called *complete proteins*. By themselves, they provide balanced protein, which the body can use to meet its own protein needs. Protein from vegetable sources are called *incomplete proteins*. They contain small amounts of one or another essential amino acid. If a particular vegetable protein is eaten by itself, the body cannot take full benefit of it as a protein source. However, by eating two or more vegetable proteins, ech of which makes up for the other's deficiencies, one can produce a complete protein. These combinations are called *complementary proteins*.

**Anemia:** A blood condition commonly called weak or thin blood caused by an insufficiency of red blood corpuscles or of the total amount of hemoglobin in the bloodstream or both. It usually is due to an iron-poor diet.

**Assimilate:** To change food into a form that can be absorbed by and made part of one's body tissues.

**Behavior:** The way one acts, reacts or functions in a particular way that can be observed. The way one conducts one's self.

**Benzedrine** A stimulant, which has a paradoxical

**(Amphetamine Sulfate):** Calming effect on the hyperactive child.

**Brewer's Yeast:** Now known as *nutritional yeast* (no longer an exclusive by-product of beer-making). It is bred to be used as a food for extra nutrients; a bountiful source of protein and the B vitamins.

**Carbohydrates:** Chief source of energy, along with fat and protein. Basically there are two kinds of carbohydrates — the *starches,* called complex carbohydrates, and the *sugars,* or simple carbohydrates. There are also *natural* carbohydrates, both simple and complex, found in foods as they come in their original form from the earth. And there are *refined* or *processed* carbohydrates, extracted from their original natural forms and added to foods (such as cakes, cookies, pies, candy, etc.).

**Constipation:** A condition in which the stools are hard and usually large and dry. Bowel elimination is infrequent and difficult, the main cause being consumption of foods low in roughage (fiber).

**Cylert (Pemoline):** A drug structurally dissimilar to amphetamines and methylphenidate, but with a pharmacological activity similar to that of other known central nervous system stimulants. Although it is a central nervous system stimulant, it has a paradoxical calming effect on the hyperactive child.

**Delinquency:** A term usually restricted to adolescent and younger children. It pertains to their failure or neglect to do what duty or the law requires. It refers to commission of aggressive, antisocial acts, such as defying authority (parental or social), refusing to attend school, running away, stealing, vanalism, speeding, arson, assault, murder, etc.

**Depression:** One of the most common illnesses. True depression is sadness plus feelings of hopelessness and inadequacy — the belief that life will not get better.

**Dexedrine (Dextroamphetamine Sulfate):** A stimulant, but has a paradoxical calming effect on the hyperactive child.

**Diarrhea:** Excessive frequency and looseness of the stool.

**Discipline:** Strict control to enforce obedience; punishment intended to correct or train, such as the training that develops one's self-control, character, orderliness, and efficiency.

**Drug Abuse:** Term applied to the use of drugs to an extent far beyond their usual medical indications. To wrongly or improperly misuse them.

**Dyslexia:** Difficulty with reading (*dys* — difficult; *lexia* — reading). Although difficulty with reading can be due to many different causes, the term usually pertains to one who has a *Specific*

*Learning Disability* (SLD). Dyslexia, then, is one of the specific learning disabilities, meaning that a person has trouble reading.

**Dysfunction:** Any abnormality or impairment of a body organ or part.

**Enzymes:** Substances produced by the body to break down food so it can be absorbed by the intestines.

**Epinephrine or Adrenalin:** A chemical secreted by the adrenal glands. Stimulates the heart, increases muscular strength and endurance, prepares the body for "fight, flight, or fright."

**Fructose:** Fruit sugar found in sweet fruits and honey; sweetest of the commonly used sweeteners.

**Gastrointestinal:** Relates to the stomach and intestines.

**Genetic:** Relates to cytogenetic, chromosomal and heredity factors, which determine one's physical and mental potential.

**Learning Disabled (LD):** Pertains to one usually considered to have near average or above-average intelligence, but experiences problems in one or more of these areas: listening, thinking, talking, reading, spelling, writing, math or remembering. Some specific learning disabilities are: Dyslexia — reading disability; Dysgraphia — writing disability; Dysorthographia — spelling disability; Dyscalculia — math disability.

**Malabsorption:** General wasting of body tissues that occurs when food passes through the intestines without being digested and/or absorbed.

**Malnutrition:** A condition resulting from an insufficient intake of food, a poorly balanced diet, defective digestion, or a defective utilization of food.

**Matabolism:** Transformation of food into basic elements for growth and energy.

**Nervous System:** A network of enormous complexity, it is a means of communication within the body and with the outside world; coordinates and controls responses to stimuli and conditions one's behavior and consciousness. The nervous system consists of the brain, spinal cord, nerves and sense receptors (sight, hearing, smell, taste buds, and numerous cells throughout the skin which relay information about pain, pressure, temperature). The central nervous system is the brain and spinal cord. The peripheral nervous system is the branching network which supplies the skin, muscles, and internal organs.

**Norepinephrine:** Related to epinephrine, a hormone excreted by the medulla or adrenal glands.

**Nutrients:** Parts of food that help the body function correctly.

**Paranoid:** Characterized by oversuspiciousness or delusions of persecution.

**Phobia:** Irrational, excessive, and persistent fear of some particular thing or situation.

**Proteins:** "Building blocks" of the body; basic food substance found in all living matter.

**Ritalin (Methylphenidate):** Nonamphetamine drug with stimulant properties similar to amphetamines. It, too, has a paradoxical calming effect on the hyperactive child.

**Schizophrenia:** Major mental disorder of unknown cause, marked by a loss of contact with reality, accompanied by delusions and hallucinations, fragmentation of the personality, motor disturbances, bizarre behavior. *Schizo* means split and *phrenia* means brain.

**Stimulus:** Anything that excites an organ or part of the body, causing it to react.

**Syndrome:** Group of signs or symptoms occurring together, characterizing a specific disease or condition.

## APPENDIX F: Suggested Reading

### Allergy

Crook, William G., M.D. *Are You Allergic?* Professional Books, P.O. Box 3494, Jackson, Tennessee 38301, 1974.

Crook, William G., M.D. *Tracking Down Hidden Food Allergy*, Professional Books, P.O. Box 3494, Jackson, Tennessee 38301, 1978.

Frazier, Claude A., M.D. *Coping With Food Allergy,* Quadrangle/The New York Times Book Co., 1974.

Frazier, Claude A., M.D. *Parent's Guide to Allergy in Children,* Grosset & Dunlap, 1973.

Gerrard, John W., D.M., F.R.C.P. *Understanding Allergies,* Charles C Thomas Publisher, 1973.

Ludeman, Kate, Ph.D. and Henderson, Louise. *Do-It-Yourself Allergy Analysis Handbook,* Keats Publishing, Inc., 1979.

Mandell, Marshall, M.D. and Scanlon, Lynne Waller. *Dr. Mandell's 5-Day Allergy Relief System,* Thomas Y. Crowell Company, 1979.

Philpott, William H., M.D. and Kalita, Dwight K., Ph.D. *Brain Allergies: The Psychonutrient Connection,* Keats Publishing, Inc., 1980.

Randolph, Theron G., M.D. and Moss, Ralph W., Ph.D. *An Alternative Approach to Allergies,* Lippincott & Crowell, Publishers, 1980.

Rapp, Doris J., M.D. *Allergies and the Hyperactive Child,* Sovereign Books, 1979.

Rapp, Doris J., M.D. *Allergies and Your Family,* Sterling Publishing Co., Inc., 1980.

Taube, E. Louis, M.D. *Food Allergy and the Allergic Patient,* Charles C Thomas Publisher, 1973.

### Diet and Behavior

Crook, William G., M.D. *Can Your Child Read? Is He Hyperactive?,* Professional Books, P.O. Box 3494, Jackson, Tennessee 38301, 1975.

Feingold, Ben F., M.D. *Why Your Child is Hyperactive,* Random House, 1974.

Finsand, Mary Jane. *Caring and Cooking for the Hyperactive Child,* Sterling Publishing Co., Inc., 1981.

Roth, June. *Cooking for Your Hyperactive Child,* Contemporary Books, Inc., 1977.

Schauss, Alexander G. *Diet, Crime and Delinquency,* Parker House, 1980.

Smith, Lendon H., M.D. *Feed Your Kids Right,* McGraw-Hill, 1979.
Smith, Lendon H., M.D. *Foods For Healthy Kids,* McGraw-Hill, 1981.
Smith, Lendon H., M.D. *Improving Your Child's Behavior Chemistry,* Prentice-Hall, Inc., 1976.
Smith, Sally L. *No Easy Answers: The Learning Disabled Child,* Bantam Books, Inc., 1979.
Stevens, George E., Stevens, Laura J., and Stoner, Rosemary B. *How to Feed Your Hyperactive Child,* Doubleday & Co., Inc., 1977.
Stevens, Laura J. and Stoner, Rosemary B., *How to Improve Your Child's Behavior Through Diet,* Doubleday, 1979.
Stewart, Mark A., M.D. and Wendkos, Sally Olds, *Raising a Hyperactive Child,* Harper & Row, 1973.
Sugarman, Gerald I. and Stone, Margaret N. *Your Hyperactive Child,* Henry Regnery Company, 1974.
Walker III, Sydney. *Help for the Hyperactive Child,* Houghton Mifflin Co., 1977.
The New York Institute for Child Development, Inc., with Richard J. Walsh. *Treating Your Hyperactive and Learning Disabled Child,* Anchor Press/Doubleday, 1979.

**Diet and Health**

Block, Zenas. *It's All on the Label,* Little, Brown and Company, 1981.
Brody, Jane E. *Jane Brody's Nutrition Book,* W. W. Norton & Company, Inc., 1981.
Bruder, Roy, Ph.D. *Discovering Natural Foods,* Woodbridge Press Publishing Company, 1982.
Campbell, Diane. *Step-By-Step to Natural Food,* CC Publishers, 1979.
Clark, Linda. *Know Your Nutrition,* Keats Publishing, Inc., 1973.
Goeltz, Judy. *The Beginner's Natural Food Guide and Cookbook,* Hawkes Publishing, Inc., 1975.
Martin, Jeanne. *For the Love of Food,* Ballantine Books, 1982.
McEntire, Patricia. *Mommy, I'm Hungry,* Cougar Books, 1982.
MacNeil, Karen. *The Book of Whole Foods: Nutrition & Cuisine,* Vintage Books, 1981.
Mindell, Earl. *Earl Mindell's Vitamin Bible for Your Kids,* Rawson, Wade Publishers, Inc., 1981.
Newbold, H. L., M.D. *Mega-Nutrients for Your Nerves,* Berkley Medallion Books, 1978.
Passwater, Richard A. *Super-Nutrition,* The Dial Press, 1975.
Reuben, David, M.D. *Everything You Always Wanted to Know about Nutrition,* Simon & Schuster, 1978.
Taub, Harald Jay. *The Health Food Shopper's Guide,* Dell Publishing Co., Inc., 1982.

## Helpful Cookbooks

Albright, Nancy. *The Rodale Cookbook,* Rodale Press, 1973.
Albright, Nancy. *Rodale's Naturally Great Foods Cookbook,* Rodale Press, 1977.
Barkie, Karen E. *Sweet and Sugarfree,* St. Martin's Press, 1982.
Claessens, Sharon. *The 20-Minute Natural Foods Cookbook,* Rodale Press, 1982.
Davis, Adelle. *Let's Cook it Right,* Signet, 1947.
Dworkin, Stan and Dworkin, Floss. *The Good Goodies: Recipes for Natural Snacks 'N' Sweets,* Rodale Press, Inc., 1974.
Farmilant, Eunice. *The Natural Foods Sweet-Tooth Cookbook,* Doubleday & Co., Inc. 1973.
Firkaly, Susan. *Into the Mouths of Babes,* Betterway Publications, Inc., 1984.
Kinderlehrer, Jane. *Confessions of a Sneaky Organic Cook,* Rodale Press, 1971.
Martin, Faye. *Naturally Delicious Desserts and Snacks,* Rodale Press, 1978.
Miller, Lani and Rodgers, Diane. *We Love Your Body,* Morse Press, Inc., 1980.
Zucker, Judi and Shari. *How to Survive Snack Attacks . . . Naturally,* Woodbridge Press, 1979.

# APPENDIX G: References

### Chapter 4. From Rock Bottom

1. Lendon Smith, M.D., *Foods For Healthy Kids* (McGraw-Hill, 1981), p. 91.

### Chapter 6. Snack, Crackle, Flop

1. William G. Crook, M.D., *Can Your Child Read? Is He Hyperactive?* (Professional Books, 1975), p. 84.
2. Lendon Smith, M.D., *Feed Your Kids Right* (McGraw-Hill, 1979), p. 188.
3. *Ibid.*

### Chapter 7. Forward Movement

1. Linda Clark, *The Handbook of Natural Remedies for Common Ailments* (The Devin-Adair Company, Inc., 1976), p. 21.
2. Linda Clark, *Let's Live,* March, 1980.
3. *Ibid.*
4. William G. Crook, M.D., *Can Your Child Read? Is He Hyperactive?* (Professional Books, 1975), p. 48.
5. Alexander Schauss, *Diet, Crime and Delinquency* (Parker House, 1980), p. 13, 14.
6. Susan Krajewski, *National Enquirer,* June 8, 1982.
7. Lendon Smith, M.D., Excerpt from *Feed Your Kids Right,* p. 10. Copyright 1979 by Lendon Smith, M.D. Used with the permission of McGraw-Hill Book Company.

### Chapter 10. Food: Friend or Foe?

1. Carl C. Markwood, M.D. *Let's Live,* August, 1982.
2. Victoria Moran, *Vegetarian Times,* October, 1982.
3. Bruce Fellman, *Prevention,* May, 1982.
4. William G. Crook, M.D., *Tracking Down Hidden Food Allergy* (Professional Books, 1978), p. 1.
5. Louis Taube, M.D., *Food Allergy and the Allergic Patient* (Charles C Thomas Publisher, 1973), p. 11.
6. Marshall Mandell, M.D. and Lynne Waller Scanlon, *Dr. Mandell's 5-Day Allergy Relief System* (Thomas Y. Crowell Company, 1979), p. 37.
7. Taube, *Food Allergy and the Allergic Patient,* p. 12.
8. Crook, *Tracking Down Hidden Food Allergy,* p. 49.
9. *Runner's World,* July, 1981.
10. Lendon Smith, M.D., *Foods For Healthy Kids* (McGraw-Hill, 1981), p. 213.

11. William G. Crook, M.D., *Are You Allergic?* (Professional Books, 1974), p. 75.
12. Doug A. Kaufman, *Let's Live*, November, 1980.
13. *Ibid.*
14. *Ibid.*
15. *Ibid.*
16. William H. Philpott, M.D. and Dwight K. Kalita, Ph.D., *Brain Allergies: The Psychonutrient Connection* (Keats Publishing, 1980). p. 31.
17. Victoria Moran, *Vegetarian Times,* October, 1982.

## Chapter 12. Our Supplement Friends

1. John Yacenda, MPH, Ph.D., *Let's Live,* October, 1981.
2. Linda Clark, *Know Your Nutrition* (Keats Publishing, Inc., 1973), p. 135.
3. *Ibid.,* p. 138.
4. *Ibid.,* p. 139.
5. Excerpt from Lendon Smith, M.D., *Feed Your Kids Right*, p. 31. Copyright 1979 by Lendon Smith, M.D. Used with the permission of McGraw-Hill Book Company.
6. Victoria Moran, *Vegetarian Times,* October, 1982.

## Chapter 13. Essential Fatty Acids

1. *Hyperactivity in Children,* Self Help Guides (published by Health Guides, 1981), p. 9.
2. *Ibid.,* p. 11.
3. *Ibid.,* p. 10.
4. *Ibid.,* p. 10.
5. Alan Donald, *Bestways,* September, 1981.

## Chapter 14. Hair Can Talk

1. Linda Clark, *Let's Live,* March, 1980.
2. Excerpt from Lendon Smith, M.D., *Foods For Healthy Kids,* p. 98. Copyright 1981 by Lendon Smith, M.D. Used with the permission of McGraw-Hill Book Company.
3. Linda Clark, *Let's Live,* March, 1980.

## Chapter 15. No One Answer

1. Mark A. Stewart, M.D. and Sally Wendkos Olds, *Raising a Hyperactive Child* (Harper & Row, Publishers, 1973), p. 31.
2. Andrew E. Skodol, M.D., *Woman's Day,* October 14, 1980.

3. Gerald I. Sugarman, M.D. and Margaret N. Stone, *Your Hyperactive Child* (Henry Regnery Company, 1974), p. 2.
4. Lendon Smith, M.D., *Health Express*, May, 1982.
5. *Ibid.*
6. *Ibid.*
7. Lendon Smith, M.D., *Improving Your Child's Behavior Chemistry*, (Prentice-Hall, Inc., 1976), pp. 37, 38.
8. *Ibid.*, p. 38.
9. Stewart and Olds, *Raising a Hyperactive Child*, p. 29.
10. *Ibid.*, p. 30.
11. *Ibid.*, p. 30.
12. Sydney Walker III, M.D., *Help for the Hyperactive Child*, (Houghton Mifflin Company, 1977), p. 7.

### Chapter 16. Smothering With Drugs

1. Stewart and Olds, *Raising a Hyperactive Child*, p. 16.
2. *Ibid.*, p. 17.
3. *Ibid.*, p. 248.
4. *Ibid.*, p. 248.

### Chapter 17. Unwind the Roller Coaster

1. Gerald I. Sugarman, M.D. and Margaret N. Stone, *Your Hyperactive Child* (Henry Regnery Company, 1974), pp. 14, 15.
2. Lendon Smith, M.D., *Food For Healthy Kids* (McGraw-Hill, 1981), p. 97.
3. Lendon Smith, M.D., *Feed Your Kids Right* (McGraw-Hill, 1979), p. 156.

### Chapter 18. Characteristic Pattern

1. Lendon Smith, M.D., *Let's Live*, December, 1978.
2. Doris J. Rapp, M.D., *Allergies and the Hyperactive Child* (Sovereign Books, 1979), p. 34.
3. Lendon Smith, M.D., *Foods For Healthy Kids* (McGraw-Hill, 1981), p. 102.
4. Gerald I. Sugarman, M.D., and Margaret N. Stone, *Your Hyperactive Child* (Henry Regnery Company, 1974), p. 12.
5. *Ibid.*, p. 18.

### Appendix A. The Natural Way Program

1. Mildred W. Walker, *Health Express*, March, 1983.

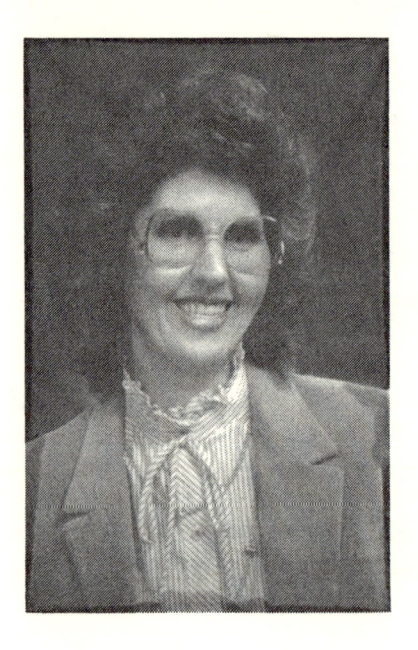

## About the Author

A native Texan, Janey Walls Mitchell now calls southern California home. Her activities include heavy emphasis on volunteer work, with her local school system for six years and as a Cub Scout den mother for two years. She is a member of the Redding, California Riders Club and a regular participant in aerobics exercise classes.

Although *Help for the Hyperactive Child* is her first book, she has written regularly for such health and fitness magazines as *Let's Live*.

# Index

Absorption of vitamins and minerals, aiding, 100-101
Acceptance, essential to self-esteem, 153
Accidents, hyperactive child vulnerable to, 155
Accomplishments, recognizing child's, 135
Additives, as allergens, 64
　chemical food, 66
Additives to avoid, 177-178
Affection, importance of physical gestures of, 159
Airola, Dr. Paavo, 198
Alcoholism, as related syndrome, 79
Alka-Seltzer Gold, to lessen allergic reactions, 78
Allergic response, immediate or delayed, 75
Allergic-Addiction Syndrome, 78
Allergies, food, may be inherited, 36
*Allergies & Your Family*, 77
*Allergies and the Hyperactive Child*, 77
Allergy, cyclic, 76
　defined, 75
　fixed, 76
　food, role in hyperactivity, 33
　role in illness, 129-130
　symptoms and clues, 79
Allowance, purpose of, 145
Amphetimines, 17
*Are You Allergic?*, 78
Attention Deficit Disorder, (ADD), defined, 111
Attention span, short, 136-137

Bad habits, breaking hyperactive child's, 144-146
Baking soda, to lessen reactions, 78
Barbados Molasses, 48
Barley malt, 48
Barnes, Dr. Broda, 127
Bedtime, setting specific, 126-127
Beef, reactions to, 59
Behavior modification, 130
Behavior therapy, 130
Benzedrine, 116
BHT (butylated hydroxytoluene), as food additive, 178
*Biological Psychiatry*, 95
Biotin, functions and sources, 189
Birthday parties, as "sugar situation", 51
Blackstrap molasses, 48
Body signs, reading, 41
Books, suggested reading, 203-204
Bowerman, Maurice, 32

Bread, adding extra nutrition to, 86
Breakfast, importance of, 89

Caffeine, as allergen, 60
　interferes with calcium absorption, 60
Caffeine habit, 87
Calcium, alternative sources, 96
　functions and sources, 192-193
　sources of supplements, 193
　supplements, 59
Calcium deficiency, 106-107
　symptoms of, 106
*Can Your Child Read? Is He Hyperactive?*, 46, 58
Carob, as allergen, 60
　as substitute for chocolate, 60
Cheese, natural, 59
Chocolate, as allergen, 59
Choline, functions and sources, 188
Chores, teaching child to help with, 145-146
Chromium, functions and sources, 193
Citrus fruits, as allergens, 61
Clark, Linda, 57
Cola, as allergen, 59
Communication, as two-way street, 159
　key to understanding, 155
Cooking tips, 169-170
Coordination, improving, 138
*Coping with Food Allergy*, 79
Copper, functions and sources, 194
　toxicity, 106
Counseling, defined, 125
Creative salads, 173-174
Criticism, need to eliminate, 159
Crook, Dr. William G., 46, 75-76, 78
Cylert, 18-19, 70, 116, 118, 120
Cytotoxic test, 81

Deaner, 18
Dexedrine, 18, 116
Diet, 30
　as treatment, 117-118
　coping with, 39-43
　importance of, 73, 114
　role in hyperactivity, 34
*Diet, Crime and Delinquency*, 59
Diet Diary, 69-73
Diet therapy, 20
Discipline, hyperactive child's need for, 157-158
　Often less effective, 157

[213]

"Diversified Rotation Diet", 76, 81
Drug therapy, advantages of, 115
Drugs, need for, 34
　role in hyperactivity, 33
　side effects, 119
　timing and dosages of, 120
Dye, red, as allergen, 75

Easy Carob Treats, 173
Educational consultant, defined, 125
Eggs, as allergens, 62
Elimination diet, 39
　diet, withdrawal symptoms on, 79
Emotional problems, as handicap, 28
　caused by hyperactivity, 30
Environment, as allergen, 63
Enzymes, role of, 100-101
Eskatrol, 17
Essential Fatty Acids, need for, 102-103
Evening primrose oil, as supplement, 103
*Everywoman's Book*, 199
Extracts, purchasing pure, 67

Fat, 107
Fat-soluble vitamins, 181
FDA, 54
*Feed Your Kids Right*, 63, 99
Feeding, importance of frequent, 88
Feingold, Dr. Ben, 54
Feingold Association, 54
Feingold Diet, 53-56
*5-Day Allergy Relief System*, 77
Fixed allergy, 77
Flour, refined, 60
　whole-wheat, 61
Food, as cause of behavior problem, 79
Food allergy, symptoms of, 74
Food families, botanical, 79
Food shopping, involving child in, 84-85
Foods, most common allergenic, 77
*Foods for Healthy Kids*, 106
Foods to avoid, list of, 173
Foods to eat, list of good, 181
Frazier, Dr. Claude A., 79
Friends, loss of because of behavior, 142
Fruit and juice concentrates, as sweeteners, 49

Gadberry, Sharon, 150
Glossary of terms, 200-203
Glucose, 51
Goals, flexible, 160
Grains, as allergens, 61
Guilt, parental feelings of, 27

Hair analysis test, (for mineral imbalance), 104-108
Hair sample, how to prepare, 105
*Handbook of Natural Remedies for Common Ailments, The*, 57
Health food stores, shopping in, 84
Health, ruling out other health problems, 124
Holidays as "sugar situation", 50
Honey, 48
　baking tip, 49
"Hyperactive" label, danger of branding child with, 161-162
Hyperactive, defined, 131
Hyperactivity, as symptom, 113
　inconsistency of, 132
　not outgrown, 115
　role in crime, 32
　role of heredity in, 112-113
Hyperkinesis, 18
Hypoactive, defined, 115
Hypoglycemia, (low blood sugar), 51-52
Hypothyroidism, symptoms of, 127

*Improving Your Child's Behavior Chemistry*, 56
Impulsiveness, 139
Independence, importance of learning, 157
Inhalants, as allergens, 75
Inositol, function and sources, 188
Insulin, control of production, 51
Iodine, functions and sources, 194
Iron, functions and sources, 194
Irritable bowel syndrome, 129

Junk foods, list of, 62

Kaiser-Permanente Medical Center, 54
Kaufman, 81
Ketchup, honey-sweetened, 68

Labels, importance of reading, 181
　reading, 65-68
Lactose intolerance, symptoms of, 57
Lead toxicity, 105
Legumes, as allergens, 61
Low blood sugar, may be inherited, 36
　symptoms of, 90
Low-carbohydrate, high protein diet, 52
Lunch swapping, 41
Lying, coping with, 148

Magnesium, 107

Magnesium, functions and sources, 195
Mandell, Dr. Marshall, 77
Manganese, functions and sources, 195
Maple Syrup, pure, 48
Milk, as cause of behavioral problems, 56
  as cause of hyperactivity, 58
  as cause of psychological symptoms, 94
  contributing to hyperactivity, 120
  excluding from diet, 56-59
  possible role in delinquency, 59
Milk intolerance, symptoms of, 57
Milk of magnesia, to lessen allergic reactions, 78
Minerals, Dr. Smith's Minimum RDA, 100
  functions of, 191
  Requirements, RDA, 191
Minerals (trace elements), need for, 190
Minimal Brain Disfunction, (MBD), defined, 111
Money, teaching child to manage, 146
Morrison, Dr. James, 115
Mother, recognizing hyperactivity, 33
MSG (Monosodium glutamate), as food additive, 178
Muscular control of speech modulation, 141
Music therapy, as outlet for energy, 150

Natural vitamins, 181
*Natural Way Program, The,* 37, 64, 94, 118
"Natural", defined, 65
Neurologist, defined, 124
Norepinephrine, 116
Nutrients, need for, 95
  requirements vary, 97, 191
Nutrition, importance of, 55
  tips, 169-170

Opthalamologist, defined, 126
Optometrist, defined, 126

PABA (Para-amino benzoic acid), functions and sources, 188
Pantothenic Acid, functions and sources, 186
Papaya enzyme tablets, 101
Parent, as coordinator of specialists, 123
Parenting, 28-30
Patience, lack of, 141
Pauling, Dr. Linus, 98
Perseverance, need for, 38
Philpott, Dr. William H., 76
Phosphate, as food additive, 178
Phosphoric acid, as food additive, 178
Phosphorus, 107
  functions and sources, 196

Potassium, functions and sources, 197
Praise, importance of, 146, 160
*Prevention,* 75
"Prevention Diet", 99
Propyl gallate, as food additive, 178
Prostaglandins, link with hyperactivity, 102
Protein, best sources, 47
  importance of, 89
Provocative test, 80
Psychiatrist, defined, 125
Psychiatry, role in hyperactivity, 33
Psychologist, defined, 125
Psychosurgery, role in hyperactivity, 33
Psychotherapy, defined, 125
Punctuality, teaching importance of, 147
Pyridoxine, (B$_6$), 94

Quick & easy recipes, 171-173
Quick treats & snacks, 167-168

Rapp, Doris H., 77
RAST, Radioallergosorbent test, 80-81
RDAs (Recommended Dietary Allowances), how they work, 99
Recipes
  Creative salads, 173-174
  Easy Carob Treats, 173
  Quick and easy recipes, 171-173
  Quick treats and snacks, 167-168
  Shakes and Smoothies, 174-176
  Tasty combinations, 168
References and footnotes, 205-208
Rejection, child's feelings of, 162
Responsibility, teaching child to assume, 147
Rewards, substitutes for sweets, 47
Rice syrup, 48
Rice, refined white, 60
Ritalin (methylphenidate) 18-19, 95, 114, 116-117
Routine, importance of, 129
Rules, hyperactive child's need for, 156-157

Salicylates, allergy or intolerance to, 178
  criticism of avoiding, 179
  drugs containing, 180
  fruits *not* containing, 179
  natural foods containing, 179
Schauss, Alexander, 59
School, 133
School phobia, symptoms of, 136
Selenium, functions and sources, 197
Self-confidence, parental, 29
Self-esteem, low, hyperactive child vulnerable to, 155

### 216  Help for the Hyperactive Child through Diet and Love

Sensitivity to foods, may be inherited, 36
Shakes and Smooothies, 174-176
Siblings, explaining hyperactivity to, 153
 often feel less loved, 154
Skin tests, 80
Skodol, Dr. Andrew, 111
Smith, Dr. Lendon, 56, 60, 63, 82, 106, 111, 131
Snacks, suggestions for, 87
Sodium, functions and sources, 197
Sodium bisulfite, as food additive, 177
Sodium nitrate and sodium nitrite, as food additives, 177
Soft drinks, best, 87
Sorghum, 48
Soybean milk, as substitute, 58
 sensitivity to, 58
Specialists, types of, 124, 126
Speech and hearing specialist, defined, 126
Sports, role in developing child's value systems, 149
Sportsmanship, poor, 141
Stealing, coping with, 148-149
Stimulants, 18
Stress, increases need for nutrients, 95
 role in gastrointestinal ailments, 128-129
 symptoms of, 128
Sugar(s), as cause of hyperactivity, 33, 46
 as filler in packaged foods, 50
 eliminating refined, 44-46
 List of Approved Substitutes, 48
 List of Forbidden, 47
Sugar snacks, danger of occasional, 46
Sugar-reward syndrome, 45
Sulfur dioxide, as food additive, 177
Summary of contributing factors in hyperactivity, 198
Summary of principles to remember, 164
Support, child's need for, 164
Synthetic vitamins, 181

Tantrums, handling, 147
Tasty combinations, 168
Teacher, cooperation of, 71
 may not recognize problem, 133-134
Techniques for raising the hyperactive child, 151-164
Television, affects on performance in school, 150
Tension, and calcium assimilation, 108
Tests, types of, 80

Thrash, Dr. Agatha M., 53, 62
Thyroid, role of in hypothyroidism, 127
Thyroid function, temperature test, 128
Toxicity, of fat-soluble vitamins, 181
*Tracking Down Hidden Food Allergy*, 76, 81
Tranquilizers, 18
Trial-and-error approach, 40
Urologist, defined, 126
USDA, labeling regulations, 67

Vitamin A, functions and sources, 182
Vitamin B-complex injections, 94
Vitamin $B_1$, functions and sources, 184
Vitamin $B_{12}$ (Cobalamin), functions and sources, 187
Vitamin $B_2$, functions and sources, 185
Vitamin $B_3$ (Niacin), functions and sources, 185
Vitamin $B_6$ (Pyridoxine), functions and sources, 186
Vitamin $B_9$ (Folic Acid), functions and sources, 187
Vitamin C (ascorbic acid), 98
 functions and sources, 189
 possible role in hyperactivity, 98
Vitamin D, 107
 functions and sources, 183
Vitamin E, functions and sources, 183
Vitamin K, functions and sources, 184
Vitamin P (citrus bioflavonoids), functions and sources, 190
Vitamins, requirements, RDA, 182
 supplements, buying, 181
 units of measure, 181
Vitamins and minerals, best sources, 100
 Dr. Smith's Minimum RDA, 99

Water-soluble vitamins, 181
Wheat, overexposure as cause of allergy, 86
 substitutes for, 86
Whole grain breads, buying, 86
Whole grains, storage tip, 61
*Why Your Child is Hyperactive*, 54

*Your Hyperactive Child*, 127

Zinc, functions and sources, 198
 need for, 103